Advance Praise for

Foundations for Clinical Neurology

"*Foundations for Clinical Neurology* is an erudite and informative book filled with the anecdotes and wisdoms of a keenly observant neurologist of vast clinical experience. It touches on many subjects of interest to the clinical neuroscientist. Dr. Laureno is widely read and has an inquisitive mind. He muses over how the ontology and phylogeny of the nervous system produces the wraparound course of the radial and peroneal nerves, how notochord remnants relate to degenerative disc disease, how bipedalism leads to meralgia paresthetica, why we hiccup and why alligators don't get dizzy. The book is filled with the clinical wisdom and aphorisms of such luminaries as Maurice Victor, Asa Wilborn, Jerome Posner, Joseph Foley, James Corbett, David Zee, Miller Fisher and Raymond Adams. I wish that Dr. Laureno had written this book years ago; I would have been a better neurologist for reading it."

—**William W. Campbell, MD**
Department of Neurology
Uniformed Services University
Bethesda, MD

"Neurologists like pearls and this book is a necklace. Each chapter is filled with helpful hints and historical notes gleaned from mentors, friends and experiences over a thoughtful career. It is both a fun and educational read."

—**Mark Hallett, MD**
Human Motor Control Section
National Institute of Neurological Disorders and Stroke
Bethesda, MD

"*Foundations for Clinical Neurology* is a satisfying immersion into the neurology culture. Laureno astutely considers the practiced approach to the patient (and flustered family) at the bedside, the subjectivity of examination, the benefits of organization, the fading eponym, the insufficient rating scales and ever changing terminology down to the single protein. Symmetry and asymmetry, disproportionality, all those crossed fibers, causality, problems in localization and how MRI has changed everything are discussed with verve. Readers will find a great exposure of the stigmata of neurology. Laureno does not shy away from iatrogenic neurology as a result of doing too much or too little. There are many remembrances of times past with omnipresent mentor musings—will we still have those tomorrow? An engaging, good-natured work that takes us beyond the traditional textbook and invites us to rethink what we do."

—**Eelco F.M. Wijdicks, MD, PhD**
Professor of Neurology
Mayo Clinic
Rochester, MN

Foundations for Clinical Neurology

Robert Laureno, MD

Departments of Neurology
Medstar Washington Hospital Center
Medstar Georgetown University Hospital
Georgetown University School of Medicine
Washington, DC

OXFORD
UNIVERSITY PRESS

OXFORD

UNIVERSITY PRESS

Oxford University Press is a department of the University of Oxford. It furthers
the University's objective of excellence in research, scholarship, and education
by publishing worldwide. Oxford is a registered trade mark of Oxford University
Press in the UK and certain other countries.

Published in the United States of America by Oxford University Press
198 Madison Avenue, New York, NY 10016, United States of America.

Library of Congress Cataloging-in-Publication Data
Names: Laureno, Robert, author.
Title: Foundations for clinical neurology / Robert Laureno.
Description: New York, NY : Oxford University Press, [2017] |
Includes bibliographical references and index.
Identifiers: LCCN 2017003948 | ISBN 9780190607166 (alk. paper)
Subjects: | MESH: Nervous System Diseases |
Neurology Classification: LCC RC346 | NLM WL 100 |
DDC 616.8—dc23 LC record available at
https://lccn.loc.gov/2017003948

This material is not intended to be, and should not be considered, a substitute for medical or other
professional advice. Treatment for the conditions described in this material is highly dependent on
the individual circumstances. And, while this material is designed to offer accurate information
with respect to the subject matter covered and to be current as of the time it was written, research
and knowledge about medical and health issues is constantly evolving and dose schedules for
medications are being revised continually, with new side effects recognized and accounted for
regularly. Readers must therefore always check the product information and clinical procedures
with the most up-to-date published product information and data sheets provided by the
manufacturers and the most recent codes of conduct and safety regulation. The publisher and the
authors make no representations or warranties to readers, express or implied, as to the accuracy or
completeness of this material. Without limiting the foregoing, the publisher and the authors make
no representations or warranties as to the accuracy or efficacy of the drug dosages mentioned in the
material. The authors and the publisher do not accept, and expressly disclaim, any responsibility
for any liability, loss or risk that may be claimed or incurred as a consequence of the use and/or
application of any of the contents of this material.

1 3 5 7 9 8 6 4 2
Printed by LSC Communications, United States of America

For Enzo, Sophie, Feynman

and

DIS • MANIBUS
Skippy

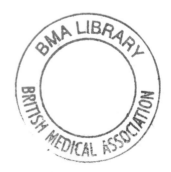

CONTENTS

ACKNOWLEDGMENTS

Thanks to the teachers who stimulated my interest in the subjects discussed in this book. At Cornell University, Dr. Perry Gilbert introduced me to the extraocular muscles and their evolution. At Cornell University Medical College, there was a rich environment for the student drawn to neurology. Drs. Fred Plum and Bernice Grafstein were among the luminaries. Dr. Jerome Posner demonstrated the complexity of neurologic diagnosis, and Dr. Paul McHugh explained the differing approaches to psychiatric diagnosis.

When I entered the residency program at Cleveland Metropolitan General Hospital, I again found a special environment. The eloquent Dr. Maurice Victor stimulated my interest in acquired metabolic diseases, symmetry, selective vulnerability, neurologic terminology, neurologic classifications, and diseases of normalization. He was a model scholar of neurology. Formative was the discipline in neuropathology provided by Dr. Betty Q. Banker. Dr. Charles "Skip" Brausch demonstrated effective communication with and practical management of patients.

Following residency, I spent happy months with Dr. Asa Wilbourn, who stimulated me to think about sensitivity, specificity, and other aspects of electrodiagnosis.

I thank the Medstar Washington Hospital Center neuroradiologists Drs. Lee Monsein, Louis Smith, Annette Virta-Paras, and Lynn Huang. Invaluable were their help with scans and their comments on the manuscript.

Mark Lin, MD, PhD was indispensable to the preparation of the book. For many hours, he adeptly assisted me with preparation of the figures, all of which are from the author or Oxford University Press unless otherwise indicated. Invaluable were the comments, suggestions and corrections of Dr. William Campbell, who carefully reviewed the entire manuscript. Drs. Mark Lin, Joseph Choi, Prerna Malla, John Lynch, Jonathan Horton, and David Zee provided helpful comments on portions of drafts. Dr. Richard Johnson kindly discussed the subject of causation with me. Mrs. Louella Baterna cheerfully prepared the manuscript in its many versions. Thanks to Ms. Jennifer Wood for library research.

Thanks also to the William B. Glew, MD, Medical Library. No librarians could have been more helpful than Mr. Frederick King, Ms. Jory Barone, Ms. Layla Heimlich, and Ms. Sharon Williams-Martinez.

Over the years, I have appreciated the help of colleagues Mr. Haile Tekle and Mrs. Marilou Wharton.

Many thanks to my Oxford University Press editors Craig Allen Panner and Emily Samulski.

INTRODUCTION

This book does not follow one of the usual formats. It is not a textbook of general neurology. It is neither a summary of neurological therapeutics nor an outline of the neurological examination. Instead, this volume discusses many topics that are not directly approached in standard texts. I hope that the student, the resident, and, perhaps, the experienced neurologist will find here something of value.

PART ONE

Practicing Neurology

1

At the Bedside

DOCTOR: "Do you drink alcohol?"
PATIENT: "No, I only drink beer."

TALKING TO PATIENTS

Patients can use a word to mean something very different from what it means to the neurologist. Once a patient told me that he had been seeing framed pictures on the wall "inverted." On a subsequent visit, I referred to his seeing things upside down. He strongly corrected me: the pictures appeared to be on the floor but they were not upside down. I had taken the word "inverted" to mean something other than what he had intended.

Communication difficulties abound. Persons of lower intelligence or lesser education may use the word "headache" for any symptom involving the head. It is common for a patient to complain of "dizziness." Only further questioning will reveal that there is no abnormal head sensation, that the real problem is imbalance. Sometimes using the patient's word can facilitate communication. The patient may say, "I feel wonky." The doctor can reply, "Tell me about the wonkiness," rather than try to translate the patient's word into a standard term.

An unsophisticated family member may use a puzzling metaphor. "She gets those dinosaur arms." Only the physician's probing reveals this image to be a reference to the small arms of *Tyrannosaurus rex*. Once we know which dinosaur she has in mind, we can understand her description of her daughter's flexed-arm ictus.

A general question about the timing of a symptom may yield little information. "Does the headache tend to occur at certain times of day?" may elicit a negative response. However, one may specifically ask whether the symptom occurs at 6 AM–9 AM, 9 AM–Noon, Noon–3 PM, 3 PM–6 PM, and so on. This questioning will occasionally bring forth positive answers for some time interval but not for others (Neil Raskin, MD, in conversation c. 1990). The elicited timing pattern may be meaningful.

Likewise, a general question about chronology may fail to elicit the critical data. If a patient states that he stopped taking a medicine shortly before a neurological event that occurred on Saturday, the neurologist will naturally ask when he stopped it. The answer may be vague. One may get different information if one asks day by day. "Did you take it on Thursday?" "No." "Did you take it on Wednesday?" "No." "Did you take it on Tuesday?" "Maybe." If one asks whether a patient smokes, she may say, "No." However, if one asks if she ever smoked, she may answer in the affirmative. When asked exactly when she stopped, the answer is occasionally, "Yesterday." The more specific questioning puts her initial answer in a different light.

General questions may not be adequate when one inquires about past medical history. A resident was called to the emergency room to consider using a thrombolytic medication on a patient with acute ischemic stroke. In the first week of his residency, he was very thorough in questioning the patient about contraindications to the drug. When she denied having a bleeding disorder, he asked whether she had hemophilia. "No." "Von Willebrand's disease?" "Yes." Again, the more specific question brought out important information when the more general question did not.

On the other hand, there are cases where the more general question brings out the critical information. A patient may not specifically remember that she has had myelitis. If one asks whether she has had "anything like a stroke" or whether she has ever had to see a neurologist, information may flow forth. It is a challenge for the examiner to sense when he should use the general question, the specific question, or both.

Distinguishing right from left is difficult for many people. The alarm of watching a stroke or a seizure does not help. A patient with old right hemiparesis may come to the hospital for a "witnessed" episode of leg shaking. Sometimes better information can come from questions that avoid the words "right" and "left." It may be helpful to ask whether the shaking occurred on the paretic side or the good side.

The doctor can be misled when patients make assumptions about their problems. One woman suffered facial ecchymosis and traumatic subarachnoid hemorrhage due to falling, which occurred when she rose from bed. "I always trip on the dog," she reported. Her husband, however, stated that the dog was not in the room at the time of the fall! Severe orthostatic hypotension was the cause of her syncope.

Families can also make assumptions. My colleague reported to me that her fiancé had high-altitude headaches whenever he went to the Himalayas on business. She wondered whether she should prescribe acetazolamide. It was eventually learned that the headaches in the Himalayas developed only in his hotel room and only in the morning when he showered before going out on business. All of the windows in the hotel's bathrooms had been sealed to keep out the cold. In each bathroom, there had been installed a small petroleum heater to produce hot water. The meaningful connection between the Himalayas and the headaches turned out to be carbon monoxide, not thin air.

Making emotional contact with a patient can help elicit information. Simmons Lessell recalled his days as a medical student at Cornell University Medical College. Aware that his supervising neurology professor was a perfectionist who was interested in psychosomatic medicine, he took an exhaustive history. The answers to his questions were not helpful. Finally, he presented the patient to Harold Woolf, the neurologist. Woolf entered the patient's room. After preliminary inquiries about her headache, its severity, duration, and location, Woolf put his arm around the lady's shoulder to sympathize, "Things aren't going too well, are they?" Whereupon she broke into tears, explaining that her son had died, that her boyfriend had run off, that she had lost her job, and that she could not pay the rent. Empathic physical contact brought an eruption of information that meticulous questioning had failed to unearth (Simmons Lessell, MD, in conversation c. 1990).

It is important to watch for patient gestures, which often provide more information than verbal responses. A patient may talk about "lightheadedness" while spinning a vertically extended index finger near his head. The gesture clearly indicates the vertiginous nature of the symptom. The same type of gesture may accompany a spoken complaint of "headache," indicating that the symptom is truly vertigo, which the patient has poorly described. A patient may report "passing out." When asked for clarification, with raised arms, he may sway side to side at the waist. It is this movement that tells the doctor that there was a vertiginous component to the episode. One patient reported that he had felt like he might faint. The examiner said, "Tell me more." The patient placed the spread fingers of a hand in front of his eyes and waved them right and left. "Why are you moving your hand?" Only then does the patient say that he had forgotten to mention that his eyes had been moving involuntarily during the episode. A patient with transient monocular visual impairment may lower his hand in front of his eye to indicate the shade-lowering visual loss of amaurosis fugax. A patient may report seeing "floaters," while his index finger draws a jagged line in the air, indicating migraine. Another, whose verbal description of a vision problem is unclear, may flutter the fingertips in front of an eye also indicating the flickering light of migraine.

For certain symptoms, it is helpful to ask a patient to demonstrate the problem. Shaking of one arm during clear consciousness may be mimicked by the patient. Sometimes the demonstration indicates more clearly that the episode was convulsive than does the patient's verbal description of "trembling." A patient may associate a symptom with a specific activity. "When I get out of bed in the morning, I step outside to smoke a cigarette and I get tingling in my legs and feet." If he is asked to demonstrate smoking, he bends his head forward and inhales as he faces the ground. The demonstration makes it clear that the symptom is that of Lhermitte. A Lhermitte symptom can also be associated with a man urinating, again because he bends his head forward to observe the process. One patient reported a funny feeling in the neck and back when she rubbed a spot on her sternum. When she was asked to demonstrate, she bent her neck to look down at her hand while rubbing her chest. The Lhermitte symptom was due to the neck flexion and had no direct relationship to her rubbing. A patient may report having headaches only when she is in the shower. She may not have noticed whether this headache occurs on bending her head forward into or backward away from the spray. When she is asked to pretend that she is showering, a head movement may become obvious.

A witness to an event may also be better able to demonstrate an episode than to describe it. When asked to "show me what it was like," a relative, friend, or co-worker may extend her arms in front of her and show fine tremors. Another might show her arms extended to her sides at 90 degrees, with large-amplitude flapping motions. Another observer may demonstrate side-to-side head shaking. Such episodes, when demonstrated, would indicate that the episode is not electrocerebral in origin. A witness, when asked about an episode she had observed, may place her finger tips at the side of the mandible and pull down that side of the face, or she may drop her arm limply, thereby indicating the nature and side of the event.

When the wife's words fail to help me distinguish a convulsion from convulsive syncope, I may ask her to demonstrate how she tried to break her husband's fall. As I go limp, mimicking the husband, she wraps her arms around me through my armpits and holds me upright. Thus I learn that the episode could have been syncopal initially. Due to the wife maintaining the patient in the upright position, the prolonged ischemia could have then led to the seizure, a convulsive component of the syncope.

For episodic phenomena, it is helpful to ask the family to make a video recording of an episode. The neurologist can then observe the event, the patient's behavior during it, and even the social setting of the event. Any of these aspects of an episode may help the physician.

There are advantages to having a spouse or some other accompanying person present when one takes the history. An obvious benefit is access to information and observations that the patient did not provide. Phone calls to a relative or witness can provide similar information when the patient has come to the clinic alone. Meeting the spouse in person can help in another way. I remember one patient who, on several visits, had reported his wife's many observations of his "abnormal" behaviors. Only when I finally met her did I learn that she was unusually attuned to every detail of her own bodily sensations. Knowing her personality helped me better judge her observations of her husband.

A patient may be voluble, flitting from topic to topic, responding to queries with a flow of information unrelated to the doctor's questions. The examiner, confused by this flood of verbiage, may suspect a neurologic problem until he questions the accompanying daughter. When the loquacious daughter responds to questions in the same way that her mother does, it becomes clear that the mother's style of speaking is a familial trait, not an acquired pathology.

It is always revealing when the spouse silently shakes his head in disagreement with a patient's statement.

On the other hand, the patient can be inhibited by the presence of the other person. He may not want to reveal personal information in his presence. Sometimes, the accompanying person dominates and offers a pressured flow of information. The patient, accustomed to this overbearing behavior, may make less effort to speak. In this situation, one can say, "I appreciate your help. First I would like to listen to the patient and then I will ask for your input."

When a patient has been sedated for a procedure, the doctor has an opportunity to interview him in a disinhibited state. The sedated patient may provide history that he had previously withheld. In fact, sodium Amytal has been given to patients for the sole purpose of facilitating diagnosis of psychiatric and neurologic disorders.

Finally, there can be multiple symptoms in one body part. For example, one person may have multiple types of headaches. They may be inexplicable and strange, but the doctor should elicit the details about each and document them as distinct problems. A patient may report 1-second stabs in the eye 3 times a year, a generalized pressure feeling in the head 24 hours a day, and a posterior head pain for 30 minutes in the morning 5 times a week. In the end, no explanation may be forthcoming for any of these headaches. On revisits, however, one may ask the patient about the first type of headache (the eye stabs), the second type (the constant pressure), and then the third type (the posterior pain). This approach allows the doctor to clearly follow the distinct types, and it communicates to the patient that the doctor has listened carefully to the patient's complaints, that he is trying to understand and help (Neil Raskin, MD, in conversation c. 1990).

GENERAL COMMENTS ON
THE NEUROLOGIC EXAMINATION

One can make important observations before the formal neurologic exam begins. If the doctor goes to greet the patient in the waiting room, he can note the patient's demeanor. He may observe with whom the patient is sitting and in what way these people interact. When the examiner meets the gowned patient in the examining room, he may note that the patient has placed 10 paper towels on the floor to avoid stepping on the tile or carpet. In a given case, such observations may be meaningful.

In general, the simpler the neurologic examination the better. If the exam is too detailed, the patient may grow fatigued, and the doctor may get lost in the details. Often it is better to use less sensitive tests to avoid finding mild "abnormalities" that are actually not pathological. Often it is most efficient to avoid quantitative methods if they are tiring or time-consuming. Having done the basic examination, one may then find it useful to selectively use a more sensitive or more quantitative test for a given aspect of the exam.

The examiner often uses his own body as a standard to help him assess a patient's functions. Doing so is routine in examining strength. Testing vibration sense is another good example. The neurologist can hold the tuning fork in his right hand against the patient's index finger, under which the examiner can press a finger of his own left hand. If the examiner feels vibration through the patient's finger after the patient no longer feels it, an abnormality has been confirmed. Confrontation hearing examination by finger rubbing can be done with the patient and doctor face to face. The examiner extends his arms widely to his side at ear level. If the examiner hears the fingers of a hand rub and the patient does not, an abnormality is present.

Our knowledge of physical findings and their meaning has developed empirically. In modern medicine, empiricism is not always respected. Today, we speak of sensitivity, specificity, reliability and validity, negative predictive value and positive predictive value. Because there has been little validation of the meaning of neurologic signs, even the most venerable can be questioned. The undertaking, however, can be difficult. First of all, patients are very different from one another. Furthermore, the circumstances of such studies can be artificial. Hence their results can be misleading.

Babinski described the plantar reflex abnormality that bears his name. All medical students learn that reflex great toe extension after appropriate stimulation of the sole indicates corticospinal tract dysfunction. What a surprise it was to open a proper journal and find an article questioning whether the plantar reflex had any use![1] The authors studied 10 patients with known "upper motor neuron dysfunction." These patients were examined by multiple doctors, including internists, family practitioners, and emergency room doctors. The interrater reliability for the presence of a Babinski sign was not as good as that for decreased speed of foot tapping. The authors suggested that testing for a Babinski sign should be deemphasized. They conceded, nevertheless, that the Babinski sign could be helpful in uncooperative patients or in patients with combined upper motor neuron and lower motor neuron disorders.

Although this comparison of tests was admirable in its statistics and its blinding (only the leg exposed), this study circumstance was not similar to neurologic practice in which the doctor is trying to determine whether or not there is a corticospinal tract disorder. Landau points out that in neurologic practice the plantar reflex must be considered in the light of the rest of the neurologic exam, particularly in comparison to the plantar reflex of the other side. Furthermore, Landau states that it is unreasonable to compare an involuntary reflex with a voluntary repetitive movement.[2] In fact, all experienced clinicians know that the Babinski sign is useful, statistics notwithstanding. Thus, Martin Samuels has succinctly and correctly stated that the findings of this study are "simply not true."[3] We must accept that the neurologic exam and its interpretation are to a large extent based on empirical knowledge.

PALPATION

Palpation of the skull is seldom needed to detect an old burr hole in our era of readily available head imaging. However, palpation remains useful to the neurologist. For certain patients, an emotional connection to the examiner can come from the laying on of hands (Gaetano Molinari, MD, in conversation, 1979). There can be great psychologic benefit to the patient who perceives that the doctor is taking the headache seriously enough to carefully (not fleetingly) examine his head.

Feeling a warm knee, ankle, and/or toe may alert the neurologist to the possibility that the "weak" leg is showing poor strength due to the pain of gout. For an older patient with headache, it is appropriate to massage the temporal artery to check for tenderness. One may ask the patient: "Does this massage make the headache better?" The neurologist's suspicion of a serious disease may be enhanced by one answer and diminished by another.

COMMENTS ON EXAMINATION OF STRENGTH

When a patient has paralysis, the "weakness" sometimes appears to be more extensive than it actually is. The misimpression can result from inadequate examination or from misleading patient behavior. Radial neuropathy is a good example of this problem.

In radial neuropathy, wrist drop occurs. With the hand in the dropped position, examination of the interossei (ulnar nerve innervated) or abductor pollicis brevis (median nerve innervated) will not demonstrate the true strength of these muscles. One might interpret this "weakness" as being outside the distribution of the radial nerve and therefore suggestive of a diagnosis other than radial neuropathy. If the examiner supports the hand in a passively dorsiflexed position, he can see the good strength of the interossei and abductor pollicis brevis and conclude that only muscles supplied by the radial nerve are affected.

Sometimes, on the other hand, it is patient behavior that makes the weakness seem to be more extensive than that expected from a radial neuropathy. A depressed patient may view his fingers as paralyzed, having repeatedly tried to use them. When the examiner tests the strength of the interossei or abductor pollicis brevis, the patient may not have the mental energy to move them; he has already "decided" that his hand is paralyzed. He has, in a sense, given up. The doctor must recognize the situation and encourage the patient to try again.

A similar phenomenon can be seen in a femoral neuropathy after hernia repair. The patient may report left leg paralysis as, "I can't move anything." The patient has generalized the weakness in his mind. He has to be coaxed out of it. Reassuringly, the doctor can say, "I know that you can't do this" (testing hip flexion). "Now don't let me push your foot down" (eliciting good dorsiflexion at the ankle).

Excess "weakness" can also be misleading when a patient is eager to seek a formal determination of disability. Trying to take advantage of a radial mononeuropathy, such a patient may demonstrate weakness of all finger movements. Similar exaggeration may occur with other mononeuropathies or after trauma. For example, a high-voltage shock to the right arm brought a patient to the hospital where, over the next day, under observation, the patient developed "weakness" of the right arm and then the right leg. The electrical trauma had been real and dangerous, but the feeble movements shown on strength testing were not due to true hemiparesis. Nevertheless, this "weakness" resulted in his "inability" to work during a long period of rest and rehabilitation. The idea that the right side of the body had been injured had been elaborated into the right "hemiparesis."

All neurologists know that gravity is important when one is grading strength in the limbs or doing a Dix-Hallpike maneuver. Gravity can also be useful to the examiner in other ways. The head-dropping test[4], for example, requires the patient to be supine. The examiner's hand cups the occiput.

Suddenly and without warning, the examiner uses his other hand to lift the head and then drop it. In a normal person, the head drops like a dead weight. In Parkinson disease, as an early sign, the head moves slowly and steadily down toward the table. Gravity can also be useful in examining a patient with ptosis, which appears less severe when the head is allowed to hang down off the examining table. "Ptosis" due to a psychiatric problem will not be improved by head hanging.

COMMENTS ON THE SENSORY EXAMINATION

On each occasion, it is best to keep the sensory exam brief to avoid patient fatigue. The sensory exam is subjective; it depends on clear communication between the examiner and the patient. The examination is soundly based when the doctor is certain that the patient understands what is being asked of him. When checking position sense, the neurologist might say, "Look at your toe. When I move it this way, it is going up. When I move it this way, it is going down." In a case where it is unclear how well the patient is grasping the idea, I ask the patient to watch while I repeatedly move the toe up or down, asking him to name each movement. Only when I am certain that we both are using the words "up" and "down" in the same way do I tell him to look away. Then I begin testing.

The use of dummy stimuli reassures the examiner that the patient's understanding, alertness, concentration, and cooperation allow for a meaningful sensory examination. Do not say, on rubbing fingers by a patient's ear, "Do you hear this?" It is better to say, "Tell me if you hear my fingers rubbing." Then one can admix no-contact (i.e., soundless) finger movement with finger rubbing stimuli to determine whether the patient actually hears. One can similarly test smell. Occluding one nostril, one can bring a piece of paper towel up to the open nostril. "Do you smell anything?" Use of this odorless stimulus can be admixed with use of a real stimulus like perfumed liquid soap on a piece of paper towel. Light touch stimuli can likewise be admixed with non-contact "stimuli." With each stimulus, one can say, "Do you feel this?"

One must select the proper stimulus to provide the most useful clinical information in a given situation. Confrontation visual field testing is a fine example. The field may be tested in four quadrants by hand movement, finger counting, or color. Depending on the situation, the less sensitive test or the more sensitive test may be most revealing. In a given case, there may be no intact field detected by finger counting. However, when hand motion is used, one may find residual vision in the nasal field in each eye. In other words, using hand motion reveals disproportionate bi-temporal hemianopia.

Demonstration of this pattern of deficit is important in localizing a disease process. In another case, a patient may have normal finger-counting visual fields. When the patient is asked to compare the intensity or sharpness of a red test object in the quadrants of vision, a homonymous hemianopia may become evident. Combining different tests improves the sensitivity of confrontation visual field testing.[5]

Selection of the proper stimulus or method of sensory testing is important in other portions of the sensory examination. A patient may hear a 512 cps tuning fork in each ear but may not hear a finger rub. A patient may not have the concentration to distinguish a pinprick from a dull touch but may be able to compare the temperature of a cold test object on one side of the body to the other. Lightly stroking the examiner's fingers against the patient's skin is a very sensitive screening test. This method stimulates many different types of nerve fibers at once. The patient can describe whether this stroking feels the same or different on the left and right sides. The patient can also report whether the stroking feels more natural proximally or distally (William Brown, MD, in conversation, 1996) or whether a tickle on the soles feels normal (William Campbell, MD, in correspondence, 2017).

In sum, there are situations in which using a stronger sensory stimulus provides the most information. In other situations, using more mild stimuli may yield meaningful results. With experience, the clinician learns to judge which approach is likely to be useful in a given circumstance.

The basic problem with the sensory exam is that concentration may fade and/or that the patient may think too long in trying to answer a question. For example, the doctor may measure the time during which the patient continues to feel the vibration of a tuning fork applied to a bony prominence. This timed vibration test is reliable in normal volunteers.[6] However, the tired, worried, or confused patient may not promptly report that vibration has stopped. He may continue to concentrate, trying to decide whether or not vibration has stopped, or he may forget the task altogether. In such patients, I avoid holding a tuning fork in place and asking the patient to concentrate long enough to tell me when vibration stops. I prefer to frequently reapply the fork, each time with a fresh question. "Is it vibrating?" "Is it still buzzing?" "Do you feel the humming?" I prepare the patient by asking him to give me a quick response to each question, to promptly answer "no" when there is any doubt and to answer "yes" only when there is unequivocal vibration. Repeating these instructions in different ways and using demonstration stimuli on the clavicle, for example, is often necessary to make the examiner confident that patient and physician understand each other. As the exam proceeds, use of sham stimuli (nonvibrating fork) can reassure the doctor that he and the patient are communicating properly.

COMMENTS ON EXAMINATION OF MENTAL STATUS

Maurice Victor taught that the heart of the mental status exam is memory testing (personal communication in conversation, 1974). He believed that one could devise his own test, a test that one finds easy and practical to apply and that gives useful information. In other words, there is no one way to do bedside memory testing. Typically, one asks the patient to remember three words or word pairs. Victor himself asked patients to remember, "Dr. Victor, Saturday, at eight o'clock." Students or residents would protest that such words could be linked together by the patient as an appointment time, that one should use three totally unrelated word pairs. Victor felt that he learned more by using his method because he was using a memory test on which any normal person should succeed: remembering an appointment. It is true that remembering unrelated words is a more difficult task and thus a more sensitive test of memory. The more difficult test, however, is more likely to be affected by the patient being worried, distracted, depressed, or exhausted. Victor, a great expert on the neurology of memory, felt that one could learn much about his patients by keeping the exam simple.

Some patients are very aware that their memory abilities are not what they once were. When the examiner tells the patient that he is going to give him three things to memorize, he may object or simply laugh, saying that he cannot remember anything. This negativism about his memory can be a self-fulfilling prophecy. To minimize this problem, I often ask the patient to remember "one thing," "Dr. Victor, Saturday, at 8 o'clock." Although there are actually three things to retain, describing them as one is less likely to intimidate the patient. In other words, describing the task as minimal can, to some extent, lessen the patient's negative thinking and thereby help him perform maximally.

When an alert patient remembers none of three test words, I sometimes return 30 or 60 minutes later. I again ask the patient if he remembers any of the words. If he now remembers two of the words, it is evident that his memory was not as bad as I had thought it was. When the patient again fails to remember any word but says, "You asked me that before, and I could not remember," I also learn something about his memory.

Occasionally, the neurologist may be entertained as he performs the mental status exam. If he is not specific in his question or directions, he may get an interesting response (Figure 1.1). Once I asked a seemingly normal patient to name the first president of the United States. "John Hanson," he answered. Recognizing my puzzlement, he explained that his ancestor had been elected president of the Continental Congress in 1781. In that capacity, he gave George Washington the country's thanks for his victory at Yorktown. On another occasion, I persisted with memory testing on a diligent patient. He was trying

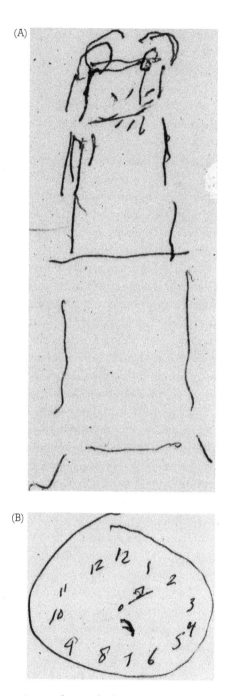

Figure 1.1 I asked the patient to draw a clock. His initial drawing caused me to suspect a neurological problem until he explained that he had been trying to draw a grandfather clock. When I then asked him to draw a "clock face," he made the second drawing.

hard and he repeatedly asked for another chance. Finally I said, "Forget it." "That's easy to do," he responded.

QUANTIFICATION OF
THE NEUROLOGIC EXAMINATION

Quantification of the neurological examination is useful for comparing examination results on one occasion to these on a later evaluation. Quantification is especially valuable in research but also can be helpful for routine clinical work.

There are different ways to quantitate the neurological exam. First, there are scored tests, such as the Mini-Mental Status Exam (MMSE). In addition, linear measurement and rating scales have been discussed as methods of quantification.[7] Quantification by time measurement is also useful. One may count the number of seconds necessary to complete a defined task, or one may count the number of repetitions of a movement or task that a patient can perform in a specified amount of time.

Of linear measurements, the diameter of the pupil is most dependent on conditions being replicable. Measurements can be compared only when ambient lighting is the same. Measurement of head circumference, on the other hand, is not dependent on ambient conditions. Comparing limb circumference is also relatively independent of circumstances. C. Miller Fisher has suggested that linear measurement is useful in measuring nystagmus excursions, limb excursions in ataxia, head excursions in titubation, excursion of the great toe in a Babinski sign, and more.[7] Such measurements have more potential for research than for routine clinical work.

All neurologists use rating scales for grading strength and stretch reflexes. The "standard" scales are neither universally accepted nor necessarily useful. The Medical Research Council scale for strength is useful for profound weakness of peripheral nerve injury and for monitoring its recovery. However, in routine clinical work, a weak muscle on this scale often falls into the 4/5 category—that is, not normal (5/5) and better than 3/5, which is power against gravity but not resistance. This British scale does not discriminate between the many gradations of power in the 4/5 range, which include slight power against gravity and resistance as well as near normal power against gravity and resistance. Many muscles correctly graded as 4/5 on this scale are severely weak. In fact, a muscle can have a 50% reduction in strength and still be graded 5/5 (Fritz Buchthal, MD, in conversation, c. 1982). Thus, this scale, invented for peripheral nerve trauma, does not work well for all cases of weakness.

C. Miller Fisher suggested that muscle strength be graded on a scale of 0 to 10, with 1 and 2 poor and good without overcoming gravity or resistance; 3 and 4 against gravity but not resistance; 5, a movement that overcomes gravity and slight resistance; 10, normal; 9, near normal; and 6, 7, and 8 gradations between 5 and 9. The group rated 4 on the British scale is thus divided into five subgroups (5–9).[7] Although Fisher solves the problem of the British scale, it may include too many divisions for neurologists to use on a daily basis. A simpler approach is to grade strength in the 4 range of the British scale as mild, moderate, or severe.

Muscle stretch reflexes are most often graded on a scale of 0–4: absent 0, decreased 1+, normal 2+, hyperactive 3+, and clonic 4+. The advantage of this system is that it is widely used and understood. Disadvantages are that many healthy people have 1+ and 3+ reflexes and that a tiny percentage of normal patients fall into that 4+ category. Nevertheless, this system can be used successfully to compare reflexes from one side of the body to the other or to compare upper and lower extremities in a given patient. Fisher's suggestion that a scale of 10 be applied (5 being normal) is too detailed to win popular acceptance. Hallett has suggested a myotatic reflex scale as follows[8,9]:

0 Reflex absent
1 Reflex small, less than normal (includes trace response or response brought out only with reinforcement)
2 Reflex in the lower half of normal range
3 Reflex in the upper half of normal range
4 Reflex enhanced (includes clonus if present)

Muscle tone can be graded as decreased, normal, or minimally, mildly, moderately, or markedly increased. A formal scale for increased tone has been proposed.[10]

Timed tests are another method of numerically monitoring patients. The patient is his own control. Documenting the time it takes a patient to walk 20 feet or to turn over three pennies on a table helps the neurologist to be more confident that a Parkinson disease patient has worsened or improved since the prior exam. How far a patient can walk in 6 minutes can be a measure of stability or worsening in multiple sclerosis and many other conditions.

Instead of a time-based test, one may count the number of repetitions a patient can perform. How far a patient can count on one deep breath is a good indicator of vital capacity at the bedside. On successive examinations, the count number may indicate stability, decline, or improvement in strength of the muscles of respiration. This test allows the neurologist to be well informed when formal tests of negative inspiratory force or vital capacity are not consistently or immediately available.

Scored tests are used mainly to quantify the mental state. This approach to bedside mental status testing became popular in the United States with the development of the MMSE.[11] This test was developed by the Folsteins and McHugh, psychiatrists. By design, this test of "mental status" excluded questions about mood, abnormal mental experiences (e.g., hallucinations), and the form of thinking. In other words, it is designed to be a test of the cognitive state in the alert patient. However, tests of language account for 8 of the 30 possible points on the MMSE. In most outlines of the neurologic examination, language is a separate category.

Alternate brief scored tests of mental status have been proposed. One test also includes language testing but has a name, the Behavioral Neurology Assessment, that indicates that it is testing more than cognitive function.[12] Another, the Short Test of Mental Status, excludes language tests, and it includes more difficult tests such as digit span and abstraction. It is a more sensitive test for cognitive dysfunction than is the MMSE.[13] Likewise, the Cognitive Capacity Screening Examination excludes language questions and puts emphasis on tests of arithmetic, opposites, and similarities.[14] The Short Blessed Test[15] was adapted by Katzman et al. from the test used by Blessed et al.[16] It is easy to use and explicitly limits itself to evaluation of "orientation-memory-concentration." Over the past decade, the Montreal Cognitive Assessment Test has enjoyed popularity. Its performance is comparable to the MMSE.[17] The Mini-Cog test has the great advantage of simplicity. It is a combination of a three-item memory test and a clock-drawing test. It seems to be as effective in the diagnosis of dementia as the longer tests.[18]

Formal psychological tests are more time-consuming. They are often proprietary. The Wechsler Adult Intelligence Scale, for example, has a long history and reputation. One must be aware, however, that documented reliability and validity of one edition is not necessarily applicable to a new version of the test.[19] In fact, it is not even clear that a new version is any better than an older one.

Coma scales have been used in the setting of cranial trauma. Because there was not a neurologist available at every emergency room that received head trauma patients, Teasdale proposed a numerical scale (Glasgow Coma Scale) for grading verbal and motor responsiveness.[20] For decades, intensive care doctors and nurses have found sequential application of the scale useful to recognize and document neurological worsening or improvement in a patient. Tracking the numbers seems less useful to many neurologists who see the scale as a great simplification of a complex neurological exam. In the 21st century, there are neurologists who specialize in critical care, and they like the idea of tracking a number but feel the need for more detail.

Wijdicks et al. have, in essence, proposed bringing more of the traditional coma exam as delineated by Plum and Posner[21] into a scale they call the Full Outline of UnResponsiveness (FOUR) score.[22] Certainly, this scoring system requires a more thorough neurological examination. The FOUR score requires that nursing personnel be much more highly trained than does the Glasgow Coma Scale. Hence, the Glasgow score can be more widely used, whereas, at very specialized units, the FOUR score can be applied. However, such units are attended by neurological physicians who can sequentially do a more thorough neurological examination than that required by the FOUR score, which does not include examination of eye movements.

Depending on the medical personnel and circumstance, it may be appropriate to monitor the neurologic exam, use the Glasgow scale for simplicity, or use the FOUR score for detailed enumeration. These are not the only scales that have been suggested,[23] but the comparison of these two scales allows us to see the benefits and problems with quantification. New scales will be proposed. Always, we must determine the ease and speed of assessment, clinical utility, and relevance to the skill level of the personnel in a given setting.

In addition to cognition and coma, scoring systems have been applied to stroke. The National Institutes of Health (NIH) Stroke Scale has been popular during recent decades. This scale was designed for research on stroke.[24] Other stroke scales exist, but the NIH Stroke·scale was used in the study that demonstrated therapeutic benefit for treatment of acute brain infarctions with tissue plasminogen activator (tPA). With the result of this study, it became essential to rapidly evaluate stroke patients for eligibility to receive tPA therapy. Consequently, it became routine for doctors to use the NIH research scale for nonresearch evaluation and monitoring of stroke patients. The American Heart Association and eventually the Joint Commission on Accreditation of Hospitals, in effect required use of this quantified neurologic examination for a hospital to be certified as delivering adequate stroke care. Thereby, the NIH scale became the dominant stroke scale. This scale has proved useful, but it is not a thorough neurological examination. For example, a patient may present with gait ataxia, vertigo, or vertical diplopia as a chief complaint of stroke. The neurologic manifestations related to these complaints may not affect the score on the NIH scale. This scale nevertheless offers consistency and speed in the evaluation of the routine stroke case.

Doctors continue to develop new scored tests for various neurologic conditions. Any of these tests may be of value to a neurologist who has familiarity with a particular test and judgment to employ it sensibly. All of these scored tests are most useful for comparing a patient's performance on one occasion to that on a prior evaluation.

REFERENCES

1. Miller TM, Johnston SC. Should the Babinski sign be part of the routine neuro-logic examination? *Neurology.* 2005;65(8):1165–1168.

2. Landau WM. Plantar reflex amusement: misuse, ruse, disuse, and abuse. *Neurology.* 2005;65(8):1150–1151.

3. Stephen CD, Saper CB, Samuels MA. Clinical case conference: a 41-year-old woman with progressive weakness and sensory loss. *Ann Neurol.* 2014;75(1):9–19.

4. Wartenberg R. *Diagnostic tests in neurology: a selection for office use.* Chicago, IL: Year Book Publishers; 1953.

5. Kerr NM, Chew SSL, Eady EK, Gamble GD, Danesh-Meyer H V. Diagnostic accu-racy of confrontation visual field tests. *Neurology.* 2010;74(15):1184–1190.

6. Botez SA, Liu G, Logigian E, Herrmann DN. Is the bedside timed vibration test reliable? *Muscle Nerve.* 2009;39(2):221–223.

7. Fisher CM. Quantitation of deficits in clinical neurology. *Trans Am Neurol Assoc.* 1969;94:263–265.

8. Hallett M. NINDS myotatic reflex scale. *Neurology.* 1993;43(12):2723.

9. Litvan I, Mangone CA, Werden W, Bueri JA, Estol, CJ, Garcea, DO, Rey RC, et al. Reliability of the NINDS Myotatic Reflex Scale. *Neurology.* 1996;47(4):969–972.

10. Bohannon RW, Smith MB. Interrater reliability of a modified Ashworth scale of muscle spasticity. *Phys Ther.* 1987;67(2):206–207.

11. Folstein MF, Folstein SE, McHugh PR. Mini-mental State. *J Psychiat Res.* 1975;12:189–198.

12. Darvesh S, Leach L, Black Se, Kaplan E, Freedman M. The Behavioral Neurology Assessment. *Can J Neurol Sci.* 2005;32:167–177.

13. Kokmen E, Smith GE, Petersen RC, Tangalos E, Ivnik RC. The short test of men-tal status. Correlations with standardized psychometric testing. *Arch Neurol.* 1991;48(7):725–728.

14. Jacobs JW, Bernhard MR, Delgado A, Strain JJ. Screening for organic mental syn-dromes in the medically ill. *Ann Intern Med.* 1977;86(1):40–46.

15. Katzman R, Brown T, Fuld P, Peck A, Schechter R, Schimmel H. Validation of a short Orientation-Memory-Concentration Test of cognitive impairment. *Am J Psychiatry.* 1983;140(6):734–739.

16. Blessed G, Tomlinson BE, Roth M. The association between quantitative measures of dementia and of senile change in the cerebral grey matter of elderly subjects. *Br J Psychiatry.* 1968;114(512):797–811.

17. Tsoi KKF, Chan JYC, Hirai HW, Wong SYS, Kwok TCY. Cognitive tests to detect demen-tia: a systematic review and meta-analysis. *JAMA Intern Med.* 2015;175(9):1450–1458.

18. Borson S, Scanlan JM, Chen P, Ganguli M. The Mini-Cog as a screen for demen-tia: validation in a population-based sample. *J Am Geriatr Soc.* 2003;51(10):1451–1454.

19. Loring DW, Bauer RM. Testing the limits: cautions and concerns regarding the new Wechsler IQ and memory scales. *Neurology.* 2010;74(8):685–690.

20. Teasdale G, Maas A, Lecky F, Manley G, Stocchetti N, Murray G. The Glasgow Coma Scale at 40 years: standing the test of time. *Lancet Neurol.* 2014;13(8):844–854.

21. Plum F, Posner JB. *The diagnosis of stupor and coma.* Philadelphia, PA: Davis; 1966.

22. Wijdicks EFM, Bamlet WR, Maramattom B V, Manno EM, McClelland RL. Validation of a new coma scale: the FOUR score. *Ann Neurol*. 2005;58(4):585–593.
23. Laureys S, Piret S, Ledoux D. Quantifying consciousness. *Lancet Neurol*. 2005;4(12):789–790.
24. Brott T, Adams HP, Olinger CP, Marler JR, Barsan WG, Biller J, Spilker J, et al. Measurements of acute cerebral infarction: a clinical examination scale. *Stroke*. 1989;20(7):864–870.

2

Imaging

For several decades, neurologists have been able to view cross-sectional images of living patients. Analogous to gross neuropathology, cross-sectional imaging displays the brain as an entire organ but does not demonstrate microscopic tissue or cellular pathology. By allowing us to view sections of brain and spinal cord in vivo, imaging has improved neurologic practice and facilitated clinical research. This chapter deals with imaging topics that are important to the neurologist. The timing of scans, the effects of gravity, and the importance of plane of section are considered. Imaging is compared to gross neuropathology, and magnetic resonance imaging (MRI) is compared to computed tomography (CT).

These two scanning methods differ. In CT scanning, an X-ray source and X-ray detectors are rotated around the head. A computer determines the radiodensities of many small cubes of tissue (voxels) and assembles them into cross-sectional images. In MRI scanning, cross-sectional images are obtained without exposing the patient to ionizing radiation. In this method, the head is placed inside a donut-shaped electromagnet. After brief "magnetization," tissue water molecules emit radio signals, which are received by detectors outside the body. A computer determines radio signal intensities for voxels of tissue and synthesizes them into cross-sectional gray-scale images. No signal can be detected from water molecules in blood because they flow out of the section so quickly (Figure 2.1).

Each of the scanning methods has strengths and weaknesses. CT scanning has several advantages. CT scans provide a simple set of axial brain sections. Much more complex is MRI, which requires the doctor to view many sets of complementary multiplanar brain sections. Another advantage of CT is that good images can be obtained in a restless patient. When a patient is moving, a good technologist can obtain CT slices at moments of relative stillness. Thus, a complete CT scan can be done with a minimum number of attempts.

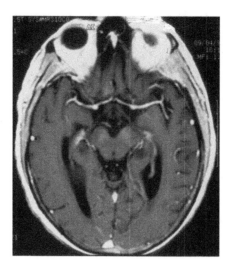

Figure 2.1 This patient died during the magnetic resonance imaging (MRI) scan.
A radiologist realized from the images on the monitor screen that the blood was not
flowing because there was bright signal from the arteries and venous sinuses.

With MRI, one obtains an entire set of slices together; patient motion degrades
the entire set of images. Furthermore, patients better tolerate CT scanning
because a CT scan can be completed much more quickly than an MRI scan.
Thus, the claustrophobic, unstable, or uncooperative patient may not be able to
finish the MRI scan, but he may be able to complete his CT scan.

In addition to these general advantages of CT scanning, there are specific
diagnostic benefits. The radiodensity of fresh intracranial blood relative to the
brain parenchyma is usually easy for any doctor to see on a CT scan. With
MRI images, fresh subarachnoid blood and tiny parenchymal hemorrhages
are less obvious and less specific in signal. CT scanning can be done when
shrapnel or other ferromagnetic materials in the head make MRI scanning
unsafe. CT scans, with their higher spatial resolution, are also better for showing the contours of foreign bodies. Although MRI scans are best for studying
bone marrow, CT scans are better for studying cortical bone, the low water
content of which impairs MRI images. Thus, CT scans are preferable for the
display of temporal bone anatomy, sinus disease, bone lesions, fractures, and
the bone–soft tissue interface. CT is likewise better than MRI scanning for
recognizing the specific densities of calcifications, gas, and intracranial or
subcutaneous fat.

The advantages of CT scanning notwithstanding, MRI is much more sensitive and specific for most brain diseases. It provides better soft tissue resolution (e.g., discriminating gray versus white matter, which have a similar

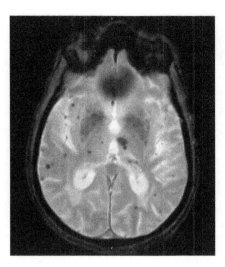

Figure 2.2 The sensitivity for blood products is shown on this gradient echo magnetic resonance imaging (MRI). None of the numerous microhemorrhages, seen on this and other slices, was detectable on careful examination at gross autopsy. Their size had been greatly exaggerated on the MRI.

shade on the black–white scale of the CT image). MRI allows us to view the brain with different sequences (i.e., different image sets, each generated by setting the MRI machine to emphasize detection of different physical properties of the tissue). The sensitivity advantage is particularly evident for small, acute lesions and for cavernous angiomas. The use of multiple MRI sequences often provides more specific information about the age of a lesion than does CT scanning. Finally, MRI can identify specific characteristics of tissue not detectable on CT scanning. Old blood product, for example, can be recognized as clearly or more clearly on MRI as it can on gross inspection of brain slices (Figure 2.2). The CT scan, however, cannot distinguish the hypodensity of an old infarction from that of an old hemorrhage.

On the other hand, artifacts are routinely encountered on MRI imaging even when there is no patient motion and no ferromagnetic foreign material. Often these artifacts are symmetric, such as those produced by normal but disparate tissue interfaces (bone–brain or bone–soft tissue). Vascular pulsation artifact also can be symmetric and can obscure the brain image. Typically, the pulsating basilar artery causes a horizontal band of distorted signal on the axial images (Figure 2.3). Extracranial metal, like dental braces, can distort the magnetic field and cause bifrontal signal abnormality. Metal-associated distortion/disruption of the magnetic field can also fail to prevent cerebrospinal fluid (CSF) signal suppression on fluid attenuated inversion recovery images

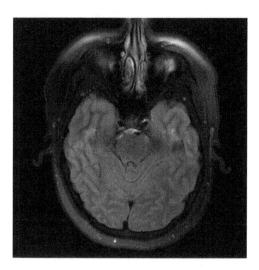

Figure 2.3 Flow from the basilar artery has caused artifact across the temporal lobes.

(FLAIR), thereby giving the appearance of subarachnoid hemorrhage. (In other words, the black CSF in the sulci is not seen.) Changes in the settings on the machine can result in misleading images. For example, incorrect settings of the time between and the duration of radiofrequency pulses can affect images.

No creative method in neuropathology can match imaging's ability to show a full set of sections in three planes, one plane better for demonstrating one disease and a different plane for another. Nutritional cerebellar degeneration of the anterior superior vermis is best demonstrated on the midline section. Optic neuritis is best displayed on coronal sections through the optic nerve. The relationship of multiple sclerosis plaques to the corpus callosum is seen optimally on sagittal images of the brain. On the other hand, the Dawson finger shape of plaques is better seen in axial and coronal sections. Of course, the bilateral symmetry of metabolic/toxic diseases is well displayed on coronal and axial cuts but is not so obvious on sagittal slices.

Plane of section is also important in spinal imaging. In a case of radiculopathy one can see a lateral lumbar disc protrusion best on axial sections. The sagittal sections are better when lumbosacral nerve root compression is due to narrowing of a neural foramen, be it by bony hypertrophy or disc, because only the sagittal sections show the entire outline of the foramen. Any axial section, due to the orientation of the foramen, can show only a portion of the outline. There is less advantage of the sagittal images in the cervical spine, where the neural foramina are angled differently.

The sensitivity of each imaging method or sequence depends on the timing of the scan. For very early subarachnoid blood, the most sensitive test is probably CT scanning; FLAIR MRI images are also very good early on. Gradient echo (GRE) images usually take a few days to show subarachnoid blood. Although diffusion-weighted imaging (DWI) is an excellent sequence to show acute infarction, it is not always the best sequence to demonstrate very early infarcts. Especially in the brainstem and thalamus, T2-weighted imaging or apparent diffusion coefficient (ADC) images can show early small infarcts when the DWI sequence does not.

The advantage of one MRI sequence over another is not limited to acute infarcts. As a generalization, T2-weighted imaging gives better resolution for brainstem lesions than does FLAIR. Conversely, the FLAIR images are better than T2-weighted images in the cerebral hemispheres.

In imaging, thinner slices that are contiguous can show disease missed by thicker noncontiguous slices. For routine purposes, it has not been practical to use these methods because they take too much time. In a specific instance, however, the clinician can request special attention to a specific territory with the more sensitive techniques. Improvements in technology will no doubt allow more routine contiguous thin-slice scanning in the future.

Gravity has long been an important factor in neuroradiology, and it continues to be important in the era of cross-sectional imaging. Most scans are performed when the patient is supine. Settling of the cauda equine is normal in the supine patient. Likewise, atrophic cerebral hemispheres settle against the inner table of the occipital bones. Thus frontal lobe atrophy is more evident than occipital lobe atrophy. Similar down-settling occurs when blood has entered the ventricular system. There results a fluid level: CSF above and blood below. Likewise, a level can occur in ventriculitis: CSF above and pus below. A ruptured dermoid cyst also can lead to a ventricular fluid level: fat above and CSF below. Fluid levels occurs under other circumstances. For example, in the presence of coagulopathy, a parenchymal brain hemorrhage, unable to clot, will develop a level, plasma above and blood cells below (Figure 2.4). A similar level can occur in head trauma, after which an air above subarachnoid CSF or air above subdural blood level can result. An air above fluid level frequently occurs in acute maxillary sinusitis.

Long before the invention of cross-sectional imaging, use of gravity was essential for neuroradiologists who performed myelography and pneumoencephalography. Having placed contrast material in the subarachnoid space, the radiologist would have the patient stand. The resulting gravitational stress on the spine would make lumbosacral root compression more evident. (Likewise, MRI scanners, which allow the patient to be scanned while he is standing, better display narrowed intervertebral foramina or lumbar disc protrusion.) Neuroradiologists were expert at somersaulting, rolling, and otherwise maneuvering patients to move air (injected by lumbar puncture)

(A)

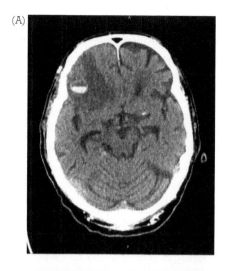

(B)

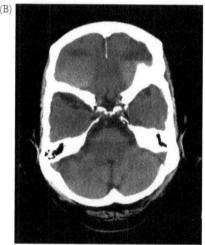

Figure 2.4 A plasma over red cell fluid level occurs when blood does not clot. The coagulopathy is typically due to anticoagulant medicine. Most often this fluid level is seen in a cerebral hemorrhage. Here, it is shown in (A) hemorrhagic infarction and in (B) subfrontal hematomas.

into parts of the ventricular system that they wanted to show on a skull X-ray. In the era of modern imaging, a patient, by changing position, may unintentionally but similarly cause an intraventricular mass (e.g., cysticercosis) to migrate in the ventricular system between the performance of a first scan and a subsequent one.

Although CT scanning and MRI scanning have transformed clinical neurology, they are not perfect. Some regions (detail of the interior of the cavernous sinus) and structures (lateral geniculate bodies) are very difficult to see well. For certain disease processes, scanning is insensitive. For example, small vessel vasculitis without brain infarcts will not be detected. Second, images do not always correlate well with symptoms. One may have excruciating headache from a CSF leak without the scan showing features characteristic of low CSF pressure. Likewise, a patient may have signs of Wernicke disease without change on the MRI scan. On the other hand, a patient with an image demonstrating brain shifting from a chronic subdural hematoma may be asymptomatic. Finally, there is often poor correlation of images with prognosis. One may have poor-outcome anoxic encephalopathy with unimpressive brain images. On the other hand, a patient with ominous looking images in diseases such as acute disseminated encephalomyelitis or pontine infarction can recover very well. Finally, an MRI sequence, designed to be sensitive to blood products, can mislead the clinician by making a cavernous angioma or microhemorrhage look much bigger than it is. In sum, our brain images are superb but imperfect laboratory tests.

There are situations when the neurologist may order a scan although the signs and symptoms do not absolutely necessitate the testing. Because noncontrast MRI scanning carries no risk of ionizing radiation or contrast allergy, such "unnecessary" testing can be done safely. One example is patient concern about family history. A patient whose father died of a subarachnoid hemorrhage may be very concerned about his headaches. Great reassurance can be provided by normal CT or MRI images of the arteries. Protecting a patient's legal interests can also make it reasonable to order images. A patient, alert after suffering a concussion, may have asymptomatic subarachnoid hemorrhage or brain contusion. Demonstration that the lesion is acute at the time of the emergency room visit documents a temporal relationship of the brain injury to an accident. Establishing this chronology may be important to the patient 10 months later, when he begins to have seizures. Evidence-based clinical guidelines may not support and payors (insurance companies) may not approve scans done for such reasons.

A few pitfalls of cross-sectional imaging deserve mention. First, when one compares an MRI scan to an image obtained on another occasion, one must be aware that the two studies may have been done on different scanners. For example, a test performed on a higher strength magnet would show more flow artifact. Second, if one orders a noncontrast scan, he can be misled by residual contrast from a prior study: for example, a chest CT exam done with contrast the previous evening. Although the brain study is performed as a noncontrast study, it is actually a contrast study. This problem is most likely to occur in a kidney failure patient due to delayed renal clearance of contrast from the circulation. Third, if an MRI noncontrast scan is done the day after an enhanced scan, the residual gadolinium may give the appearance of subarachnoid blood over the surface of a cerebral infarction with disrupted blood–brain barrier. Finally, one can be confused by superimposition of an acute process on an old lesion. On FLAIR images, the area of increased signal due to an old infarct may be contiguous with an area of increased signal due to postictal "edema." With treatment of the seizures and passage of time, the postictal change clears and a repeat scan shows the limited extent of the original lesion.

We have learned a lot about neurologic disease from cross-sectional brain imaging. For example, the intracranial correlates of low CSF pressure headache became evident with MRI scanning. Never witnessed by a pathologist but obvious to the radiologist are the venous dilatation, the dural thickening, the change in chiasmal position, and the cerebellar tonsillar herniation in many cases. Rarely seen by a pathologist, the lesions of Bell's palsy are nicely seen on MRI scans. Sequential scans have helped us study the gradual enlargement of brain hemorrhages and the timing of hemorrhagic transformation of embolic infarctions. Furthermore, sequential scans have demonstrated the cure by antibiotics of multiple brain abscesses in tuberculosis and bacterial disease. In addition, sequential images in cases of hypertensive encephalopathy made evident the associated areas of focal brain edema that resolve with treatment of hypertension. These are a few examples of advances in knowledge brought by MRI. Prior to sequential imaging, sketchy knowledge of these subjects came through observations of autopsy series. With imaging, these changes can be better observed in individual patients.

Sequential imaging is also a fine tool for the study of experimental disease. For example, the acute lesions of experimental allergic encephalomyelitis can be visualized repeatedly over days. Performing autopsies of groups of animals at different intervals allows correlation of the sequential images with the changing microscopic features of the lesions.

Finally, MRI scanning has not only taught us about disease. It has informed us about normal neurology such as developmental myelination of the brain Easily seen on MRI is extraocular muscle enhancement, which provides one more clue to the special nature of these muscles. Other skeletal muscles do not enhance.

Reviewing the history of neuroradiology helps one appreciate the stunning advance brought by computerized, cross-sectional imaging. In the past, X-rays and then X-ray tomograms provided information about bony features like hyperostosis, erosion of bone, and enlargement of the sella turcica. With the advent of ventriculography and especially pneumoencephalography, the CSF space was visualized. Later, intra-arterial injection of radiodense contrast media allowed us to see the course and contours of the lumens of the cervical and cranial vasculature. A further advance came with intravenous injection of radioactive isotopes, which allowed demonstration of areas of blood–brain barrier breakdown (nuclear "brain" scans). Today, both CT and MRI scanning allow us to see bone, CSF space, arteries, veins, blood–brain barrier breakdown, and the brain itself. Doctors entering practice in the 21st century cannot easily understand how neurology was practiced before the advent of cross-sectional imaging.

As technology progresses, scanning methods will change. The basic concepts, however, will stand. To most effectively interpret cross-sectional imaging, the neurologist will always have to consider the plane of section, the timing of scans, the timing of clinical events, the effects of gravity, and the strengths and weakness of the various imaging methods.

3

Diagnosis

All diagnostic tests have limitations. The electroencephalogram is not always abnormal in epilepsy. Cerebral angiography gives a beautiful display but cannot show small vessel vasculitis. Brain magnetic resonance imaging (MRI) is not perfectly sensitive; it may be normal when there is obvious encephalitis. Furthermore, test results are not perfectly specific. On electromyography, fasciculations are not specific for disease. They may be benign. On the other hand, fibrillations, always pathologic, are not specific as to cause. They may result from primary disease of either nerve cell, nerve, or muscle. Thus, all test findings must be interpreted in their context.

Always, a diagnostic test is a sample. One may be sampling by location and/or time. Success in detecting abnormality may depend on the volume or duration of the sample. Hence, there is value in repeated or prolonged electroencephalograms (EEGs) to seek epileptiform activity. Likewise, repeated or prolonged recording of the electrocardiogram enhances detection of arrhythmia, which could be the cause of syncope or cerebral embolism. The interval between fasciculations varies greatly from patient to patient or muscle to muscle. Hence, if a needle is left in a spot for less than 90 seconds, fasciculations can be missed. Cerebrospinal fluid (CSF) testing is more sensitive when larger volumes and repeated samples are collected. One lumbar tap is often not sufficient for the diagnosis of meningeal carcinomatosis. Muscle biopsy is not a very sensitive test for polymyositis; the small sample taken may miss the patchy disease. Sural nerve biopsy has similar limitations. Likewise, a temporal artery biopsy provides a limited sample of tissue. Its sensitivity is enhanced when more numerous sections of the specimen are studied microscopically.

One can erroneously correlate diagnostic tests results with signs and symptoms. A common mistake is the association of an imaging finding, which is clearly old, with clinical events, which are current. This mistake is more likely to occur when the imaging finding is striking. For example, a patient with acute vertigo may have remarkably extensive cerebellar calcifications. The emergency room doctor may be tempted to tie the images to the clinical problem. More than once a patient with no electrolyte derangement has been found on imaging to have clearly old central pontine myelinolysis (CPM). The authors conclude from such a case that CPM can occur in the absence of a serum sodium derangement. There is, however, no telling what sodium problem may have been present when the myelinolysis, now cavitated, occurred. Such cases are sometimes published.[1] This type of difficulty in clinico-radiologic correlation is really a lack of clear thinking about the chronology of clinical events and images.

In electromyography, however, the difficulty in correlating test results with clinical symptoms is fundamentally a problem in pathophysiology. Asa Wilbourn described the problem in radiculopathy:

> The time-dependence of the EMG examination is very frustrating, and much of it is inherent to the study so it is not amenable to alterations in electromyographer behavior. This time-dependency stems from the fact that finding fibrillation potentials on NEE (needle examination) in the appropriate myotome distribution remains the most sensitive electrodiagnostic procedure for disclosing radiculopathies, and these fibrillation potentials can go undetected if the NEE (needle examination) is performed either too soon after lesion onset, before they have had time to develop, or too late, after sufficient time has passed for them to disappear, via reinnervation.[2]

ORDERING TESTS

Whenever there is a communication problem with a patient, the physician should adjust his threshold for ordering diagnostic tests. When the patient is mentally retarded, demented, withdrawn, aphasic, deaf, or not fluent in the examiner's language, nuances of history may be missed. It is better, under such circumstances, to order a scan for a complaint of headache than it is to rely too heavily on the history and physical examination. It is better to order "too many" scans rather than too few.

There are cases where the patient has no complaint or abnormality on the exam, but the spouse is concerned about a change he has noticed. In one instance, a doctor had noticed a change in his spouse's handwriting. The patient had no concern. The neurologic exam was normal. I saw no need to order imaging. Nevertheless, the patient's spouse, the physician, ordered an MRI scan, which revealed an anaplastic glioma (Figure 3.1). Repeat neurologic

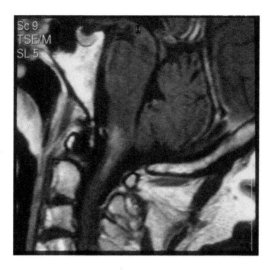

Figure 3.1 This asymptomatic patient had a normal neurologic examination. At autopsy, the brainstem lesion was an anaplastic glioma. The scan was ordered because the patient's spouse (not the patient) had noticed that the patient's handwriting had changed.

exam was normal. Always it is important to take seriously any observation made by the family.

Sometimes diagnostic tests are useful to buttress the patient's confidence in his medical evaluation. An experienced neurologist may be fairly sure that a patient has amyotrophic lateral sclerosis in a matter of minutes. However, one cannot, after a single office visit, abruptly tell a patient this terrible diagnosis. One must go through a process so that the patient can accept the grave diagnosis as legitimate. Spinal MRI scans, electromyograms, and other tests give a patient the sense that the doctor has been thorough and thoughtful rather than impulsive in offering bad news. Furthermore, following completion of these tests, the doctor has an opportunity to confirm his clinical observations before discussing his conclusion with the patient.

In deciding whether to order a diagnostic test, one must take into account the clinical context. The headache may be mild and the neurologic exam may be normal, but, if the patient is taking immunosuppressive or anticoagulant medicine, it may be prudent to order brain imaging. Subjective leg weakness in a breast cancer patient, a normal neurologic exam notwithstanding, may suggest the possibility of metastasis and early spinal cord compression. Diagnostic tests or at least an early revisit to the neurologist must be arranged. In deciding whether to order diagnostic tests, one must always think about the worst-case scenario.

Lumbar puncture illustrates two fundamental facts about diagnostic tests. First is the need to weigh the risks of the procedure against its benefits. Second, the risk–benefit calculation changes as new neurologic knowledge and diagnostic tools emerge. The common risk of lumbar puncture is low-pressure headache. The main rare but serious risks are epidural hematoma or meningitis. For more than a century, the spinal tap has been a basic tool in neurology. Yet there are little data on what precautions should be taken before proceeding with puncture.[3] Clinical experience and judgment are often the guide to weighing risks and benefits. The second topic is the changing role for lumbar puncture. At one time, spinal tap was done routinely for most patients with strokes and seizures and for all patients with multiple sclerosis. MRI has diminished the need for many of these lumbar punctures. The data are sparse. In which strokes should one seek syphilitic meningitis as the cause? In which cases of multifocal brain lesions should one examine the CSF to strengthen a diagnosis of multiple sclerosis? In which confused patients should the spinal fluid be studied for infection? It is often clinical experience and judgment that determine whether or not it is wise to perform lumbar puncture or other diagnostic tests.

DIAGNOSTIC CRITERIA

Foremost of all diagnostic criteria are those for rheumatic fever. Jones proposed them to help with diagnosis and to minimize overdiagnosis.[4] For nearly three-quarters of a century, they have been a mainstay. There is no pathognomic sign or symptom or test that can make the diagnosis. To this day, the diagnosis of rheumatic fever is made from a list of major and minor manifestations As useful as the Jones criteria have been, strict adherence to them is not encouraged (Special Writing Group).[5] Isolated chorea is one of the major exceptions, in which the diagnosis of rheumatic fever can be made without meeting the ordinary criteria.

When rheumatic fever is diagnosed, there are implications for therapy. In other words, diagnosing the disease is tantamount to saying that the probability of rheumatic fever is high enough to justify treatment. When there is no treatment for a disease, criteria are more useful to decide which patients match a clinical syndrome well enough to be included for research on the condition. For lack of other criteria, such research criteria often are applied by clinicians in a nonresearch setting.

The formalization of diagnostic criteria for a disease is problematic. When criteria are developed by consensus of a group, they become a legislative as much as a scientific document. In addition, criteria-based diagnosis can result in the same diagnosis being applied to heterogeneous patient populations. Sometimes great energy is expended in developing criteria for a condition that is later voted out of existence. Furthermore, criteria cannot be static; they must evolve to accommodate advances in knowledge and technology.

When the criteria are formulated as lists of major features and minor features (i.e., diagnosis by two major features or one major feature plus two minor features), the criteria limit casual overdiagnosis. However, in tuberous sclerosis, for example, the patients who qualify for the diagnosis do not comprise a uniform clinical group. One applies the same diagnosis to a patient with cortical tubers and a subependymal nodule as one does to a patient with hypomelanotic macules, renal cysts, and dental enamel pits. Clinical heterogenicity persists when modernized diagnostic criteria for tuberous sclerosis are used. Now, a pathogenic mutation for TSC1 or TSC2 protein, identified from DNA of normal tissue, establishes the diagnosis independent of clinical criteria. Up to 25% of tuberous sclerosis patients, however, have no such mutation and are diagnosed by clinical criteria.[6]

Diagnostic criteria can lead to confusion. Alzheimer disease (AD) was originally a clinicopathologic syndrome. Diagnosing the entity without access to biopsy or autopsy became a challenge. As a result, criteria for clinical diagnosis were developed.

Later the concept of minimal cognitive impairment (MCI) was developed. This term was applied to persons with cognitive impairment in only one domain (memory) and with no impairment of functional activities. Subsequently, the definition of MCI was changed to include patients with deficits in more than one cognitive domain.

In 2011, revised criteria for MCI, AD, and preclinical AD were published by a working group convened by the National Institute on Aging. The revised criteria for MCI relaxed the definition of functional independence, which had been the last remaining distinction between MCI and AD. The effect, according to Morris, was to have overlapping criteria. Some patients formerly meeting criteria for AD can now be classified as MCI. "The categorical distinction between MCI and the milder stages of AD dementia has been compromised by the revised criteria."[7] Conflicting or overlapping criteria indicate a problem with the concepts, one that can be resolved only when groups can be distinguished by pathology, prognosis, or response to therapy.

Diagnostic criteria for Asperger syndrome have also been problematic. In 1994 the fourth edition of the *Diagnostic and Statistical Manual* (DSM-IV) of the American Psychiatric Association set diagnostic criteria for Asperger syndrome. The criteria were so restrictive that hardly any patient met them. The appropriateness of these criteria were less debated after the DSM-5 abolished the syndrome! In this DSM revision, all patients with autistic symptoms are placed under the umbrella, "Autism Spectrum Disorders." The change has been upsetting to families of those who have carried the Asperger diagnosis. Although the new manual eliminates the diagnosis of Asperger syndrome, it solidifies the notion of autism as a disorder. Formalizing autism as a disorder is contrary to Isabelle Rapin's long-standing teaching that autism is a symptom or finding like dementia, not a specific diagnosis into itself: "Autism is a syndrome, not a disease in the sense that measles or sickle cell anemia is a disease, because despite its salient behavioral phenotype it lacks a unique etiology or specific pathology."[8]

One investigative or consensus group may propose disease criteria that differ from those set by another committee. When there are competing criteria, neurologists try to determine which set are the "best." Typically, disagreement about diagnostic criteria occurs when there is no histologic or other specific diagnostic test available. One group looked at three sets of criteria for corticobasal ganglionic degeneration. They studied only patients who eventually met diagnostic criteria by all three sets of criteria. The authors then retrospectively examined the early neurologic records on the same patients to see which set was best at making the diagnosis at the early stage of illness.[9] As there was no pathologic confirmation in this commendable effort, the disease process or the appropriateness of diagnostic criteria were not clarified by it. Formal criteria for diagnosis of other brain degenerations have been proposed. The undertaking is problematic because these conditions have overlapping pathologies and manifestations.

In another study, diagnostic criteria for inclusion body myositis (IBM) were reviewed.[9] Twelve competing sets of diagnostic criteria had been proposed by individual authors or consensus groups. The 12 approaches to diagnosis were compared retrospectively to the "gold standard of clinical diagnosis by treating clinicians." No independent review of biopsy slides was made. One would think that meeting clinicopathologic criteria would be the gold standard rather than the opinion of the treating doctors.[10]

The 1990 American College of Rheumatology (ACR) document on giant cell arteritis requires three of five listed criteria to make the diagnosis. This guideline allows the diagnosis for an elderly man who has a high sedimentation rate and headache, a syndrome which is not specific. Such a patient might have occult meningitis. On the other hand, many biopsy-proved patients do not meet the criteria.[11] For example, the criteria disallow the diagnosis in a patient who does not meet three of the five criteria, even if he has acute monocular visual loss and a temporal artery biopsy showing necrotizing vasculitis.[11] The ACR criteria may have been good for determining which patients should be enrolled in a study; however, judgment must be used in relying on such criteria for the management of a specific patient.

Attention deficit-hyperactivity disorder is well known to the public as ADHD. Less well known is that the criteria for making this diagnosis vary from one "authority" to another. In DSM-IV (2000) and DSM-5 (2013), six from a list of nine symptoms were needed for a diagnosis of inattention. The International Classification of Diseases (ICD-10) bases diagnosis on a list of five symptoms of inattention, of which three are needed.[12] Furthermore, some doctors seriously question the entire concept of ADHD.[13] Conflicting diagnostic criteria more easily emerge when the entity is itself in question. Variance in application of criteria is another problem. The diagnostic prevalence of ADHD in 2007 was 13.08–15.52% in Ohio but 5.6–7.1% in Illinois.[14] It is doubtful that this difference represents a real biologic difference in the populations of the two states.

Diagnostic criteria evolve with technology. In recent decades, MRI has been incorporated into diagnostic criteria. Imaging best helps as a criterion for the diagnosis of a clearly defined clinicopathologic entity like multiple sclerosis. Its utility as a diagnostic criterion is less clear in degenerative disease. Some have tried to use it in diagnosing multiple system atrophy.[15]

MULTIPLE DIAGNOSES

The simultaneous presence of multiple neurologic diagnoses in one patient can be challenging (Figures 3.2 and 3.3). Sometimes two diseases or signs can occur in the same body part. Sometimes old findings may confuse the clinician who is analyzing an acute illness. Sometimes one disease can contribute to the development of another, but the clinician mistakenly tries to synthesize all the findings as manifestations of the initial condition.

A symptom can have a multiple causes in one patient. I remember an individual with a cerebral metastasis. Dizziness was the chief complaint. He simultaneously had orthostatic hypotension (too much antihypertensive medication), benign paroxysmal positional vertigo, and lightheadedness due to high doses of gabapentin and meclizine. The metastasis was not contributing to the dizziness at all. An epileptic woman whom I knew well presented with new gait ataxia. In her blood there was a phenytoin level above the usually therapeutic range, a common cause of gait ataxia. The main problem, however, was severe hypothyroidism, which can also cause gait ataxia. In another patient, headache was the chief complaint. It was attributed to the acute maxillary sinusitis seen on his maxillo-facial computed tomography (CT) scan. A subsequent CT head scan showed a subdural hematoma that proved to be an equally important cause of his headache.

A case of right-hand twitching is a good example of two conditions being responsible for a single complaint. A patient with uremia had an old left

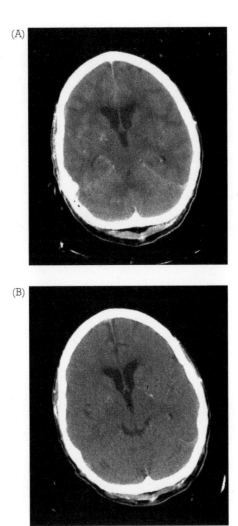

Figure 3.2 This encephalopathic patient had two causes of encephalopathy simultaneously. Extreme hypercarbia and brain swelling (A) were relieved by artificial ventilation (B), but the encephalopathy was not. Lumbar puncture revealed bacterial meningitis.

cerebral infarct, from which there had been a complete recovery. Neurologic consultation was requested for right upper extremity twitching. On my first visit to his hospital room, I found unilateral asterixis at the right wrist due to the combined metabolic and structural problems.[16] I was confident of my diagnosis. When I returned on the next day, I saw an obvious focal motor seizure of the right wrist and face, also due to the old infarct. Two types of right upper extremity "twitching" were occurring in the same patient.

(A)

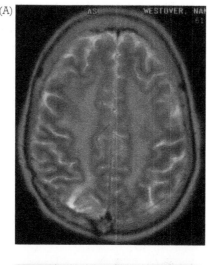

(B)

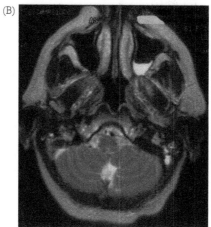

Figure 3.3 When this cancer patient complained of headache, the oncologist suspected metastasis. The radiologist's report emphasized the absence of metastases and the presence of impressive "radiation changes" in the cerebral white matter (A). The neurology consultant recognized that the headache was being caused by acute bacterial sinusitis (B). Initially, the concern for metastases and the evident leukoencephalopathy had attracted all of the attention.

When the neurologist is evaluating a complaint or illness, he may detect an old abnormality on the neurologic exam. An error may result if the neurologist attempts to synthesize the new symptom and the old abnormality. A Horner's syndrome present but asymptomatic may have been present since trauma 20 years earlier. Today's complaint of headache, taken with Horner's syndrome, may direct the doctor's thinking one way. Whereas, if its chronicity is known from review of old records, study of old photographs, or interviews with relatives, the doctor may analyze the case differently. This potential for confusion by an old abnormality occurs with many findings, including preexisting Babinski signs, hemifacial weakness, mild mental retardation, medication-induced vestibular dysfunction, and mild heredofamilial poly-neuropathy (unrecognized by the patient).

There are many examples of an old diagnosis interfering with a new one. A woman was admitted with obtundation. She had been "cross-eyed" since childhood. Initially, physicians considered her dysconjugate eyes to be a sep-arate problem from her mental state. Belatedly, it was realized that she had Wernicke disease: bilateral abducens nerve paresis had been superimposed on her strabismus. Once I encountered a patient with hydrocephalus, known since childhood. Initially, her current papilledema had been attributed to her old hydrocephalus. In fact, the obese woman had developed a superimposed idiopathic intracranial hypertension.

Sometimes one disease can contribute to the development of another (Figure 3.4). An unknown dural metastasis can present as a subdural hematoma after a minor head injury. Myopathy can cause dysphagia that can, in turn, cause nutritional deficiency. In this setting, when the neurologist encounters the ophthalmoplegia of Wernicke disease, he may, by the law of parsimony, try to synthesize the eye movement abnormality with the dysphagia.

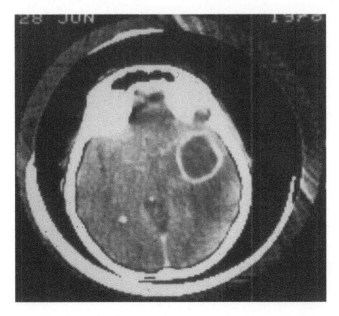

Figure 3.4 This lesion is an infected brain metastasis. Bacterial infection can also occur in a cerebral hemorrhage or a subdural hemorrhage.

The attribution of symptoms of a second disease to a psychiatric problem frequently causes diagnostic error:

A depressed janitor was found to have a squamous cell carcinoma of the pharynx, and radiotherapy was administered. Six months later, recurrent tumor was documented by biopsy. One month after this biopsy, he reported trouble swallowing and opening his mouth. After intravenous infusion of benzodiazepine medicine, the otolaryngologist easily opened the mouth, thus excluding a "frozen jaw." Endoscopy showed no obstructive mass in the throat. The patient admitted to depression and requested psychiatric consultation about his situation. The psychiatrist confirmed the presence of anxiety, depression, and conversion disorder with trismus. Two days later, he worsened to the extent that the diagnosis of tetanus became obvious.

Although depression was present, and although there was no obstructive mass or frozen jaw, it was incorrect to conclude that the dysphagia and trismus were caused by the depression.

On the other hand, a finding may be assumed to be due to a serious neurologic problem when it is actually due to a functional problem:

A patient who had experienced many well-documented bouts of idiopathic intracranial hypertension came to the emergency room. The chief complaint was headache. There was recurrent papilledema. Due to poor abduction of each eye, bilateral abducens palsy was diagnosed. Severely increased intracranial pressure was suspected. The clinicians felt a sense of urgency about the patient, who underwent multiple lumbar punctures. The CSF pressure was high. Prednisone and acetazolamide were prescribed. Eventually, however, a neuro-ophthalmologist realized that there was convergence spasm, rather than weakness of the sixth cranial nerves.

OTHER PITFALLS IN DIAGNOSIS

The circumstances in which neurologic symptoms emerge can suggest that the problem is not medical. Many young neurologists stumble in such a situation. The following case is an example:

Helen was a retired psychiatric nurse who arrived one evening in the emergency department saying that she could not move her legs. She was calm as she explained that the painless paralysis developed while she was watching a news story on Governor George Wallace, who had become paraplegic after being shot in the back. Discovering she could not walk, she somehow was able to go to bed that night and arrived at the emergency department the next day with a neatly packed suitcase. On examination she had normal muscle tone in the legs, but with effort she could barely lift her feet off the bed. All her test results were normal.[17]

Initially, the paralysis was considered "hysterical." Eventually, it was realized that the paralysis was due to anterior spinal artery occlusion.

Whenever possible, the diagnosis of a nonmedically caused neurologic disorder should be based on positive signs.[18] In the absence of such findings, the diagnosis of a nonmedical neurologic problem should be based on the collected medical data and sequential clinical observations. It should not be based on the patient's personality, psychological stress, or the circumstances at the moment of symptoms' onset.

There is potential for error whenever one feels that he is being pestered by an annoying family or persistent patient. In this situation, it is critical for the doctor get control of himself. The more "difficult" a family seems to be, the more one should reassess the patient, being careful that one's vision of a case is not distorted by one's annoyance. Difficult relatives, like pleasant relatives, make important observations. Likewise, behavior that is emotional or even histrionic should not deter one from considering serious disease as the cause of a patient's symptoms.

Knowing a patient very well can be a problem or an advantage. One can overlook a critical change if one slips into the thinking that the current hospital admission is simply the latest of many inpatient stays with similar complaints. One must always be on guard to avoid this lack of rigor. On each visit, each admission, one must freshly evaluate the patient's symptoms for intercedent factors. On the other hand, knowing a patient very well for years can be a great advantage, enabling the neurologist to instantly notice a subtle personality change that a doctor, fresh to the case, could never recognize as abnormal.

Seeing a patient in a less urgent setting can be a problem. A neurologist may be asked to check a patient for mild confusion and drowsiness. If the patient has been hospitalized for 2 months, awaiting transfer to a nursing home, the consultant may not as urgently check for hypoglycemia as he would had he seen the patient in the emergency room. It is beneficial for the neurologist to carry a little anxiety with him into environments where there is no anxiety in the air.

MULTIDIMENSIONAL DIAGNOSIS

In 1928, the American Heart Association recommended a multidimensional system for the diagnosis of heart disease listing the anatomy, physiology, etiology, and functional level of each case.[19]

For example, a patient might have a cardiac diagnosis as follows:

Anatomy: Mitral stenosis
Physiology: Atrial fibrillation
Etiology: Rheumatic heart disease
Functional state: Asymptomatic

I have often copied this approach for epilepsy patients. This method of diagnosis documentation paints a clear picture for another doctor who reads my note. For example, one might characterize the patient as follows:

Anatomy: Left temporal lobe infarction (CT head scan 2004)
Physiology: Left temporal sharp waves (2004)
Etiology: Cardiogenic embolus
Function: Government lawyer. No seizures for years

Depending on the nature of one's practice, one may use a different system of multidimensional diagnosis. Lüders, an epileptologist, uses three categories: [20]

1. Semiology of seizures
2. Etiology of epilepsy
3. Localization of the epileptogenic zone.

This approach to multidimensional epileptology diagnosis is much simpler than schemes that other seizure specialists have proposed.[20]

PROBLEMS IN LOCALIZATION

Although localizing a neurologic problem is central to diagnosis, localization is not always straightforward. All neurologists know that generalized processes can present as a focal neurologic disorder; for example, focal status epilepticus can be the first manifestation of severe hyperglycemia. Neurologists also know that a focal brain disease can present as a generalized confusional state without localizing signs; nondominant parietal lobe and fusiform calcarine hemorrhage are examples.[21]

Usually the neurologist has no difficulty in distinguishing central nervous system (CNS) from peripheral nervous (PNS) disease. However, there are situations which can be disorienting. Hypophosphatemia can simultaneously cause encephalopathy and reversible weakness due to polyneuropathy. Thiamine deficiency may cause polyneuropathy (beriberi) and Wernicke disease simultaneously. Vitamin B$_{12}$ deficiency can cause polyneuropathy dementia and subacute combined degeneration of the spinal cord at the same time. Likewise, paraneoplastic disease can cause peripheral weakness and cerebellar degeneration in the same patient. In such instances, the neurologist must recognize the simultaneous occurrence of CNS and PNS disease and think of the possible explanations.

Likewise, neurologists attempt to systematically categorize a neuromuscular condition. Is the weakness due to a disorder of nerve, neuromuscular junction, or muscle? Diseases do not always conform to this simple classification. Thus one patient with proximal weakness turned out to have a combination of myositis and myasthenia gravis, both of which responded well to prednisone treatment. Another patient had both stiff person syndrome and myasthenia gravis. Patients have been reported to have both myasthenia gravis and Eaton-Lambert syndrome.[22] In cancer patients, there can occasionally occur a combined neuromyositis. Colchicine toxicity is well known to cause neuromyopathy.

FINAL COMMENTS

1. In trauma patients the neurologist can be misled in different ways. If a patient enters the hospital with major trauma, the neurologist may detect an abnormality that is not necessarily due to that trauma. The stiff neck may have been there before the child fell off the tricycle. After an automobile accident, the doctor may be called to evaluate a patient for seizures. He should always consider the possibility that a seizure caused the accident rather than assume that the seizures are consequent to the trauma. When there is no history of trauma, on the other hand, remember that a neurologic abnormality actually may be due to trauma that the patient has forgotten or has chosen not to mention.

2. Diagnosing the cause of pain can be challenging. Although distractibility is useful in diagnosing a movement disorder as "psychogenic" (nonmedical cause), distractibility from pain should not be used to support a diagnosis that pain is nonmedical. In fact, one should never diagnose pain as nonmedical (Joseph Foley, MD, in conversation, 1975).

3. Recognition of urgency is as important in diagnosis as localizing a process and determining its cause. Severe hydrocephalus that has obliterated the subarachnoid space around the brainstem is an example. Although the patient may be alert and totally clear-minded, one cough can lead to brainstem compression and respiratory arrest.[23] The neurologist must not be reassured by the patient's normal mental state. He must call for immediate surgical intervention. This is one of many situations in which the neurologist must recognize urgency and act.

4. Increased use of a diagnosis does not necessarily indicate increased occurrence of a disorder. Diagnostic expansion, diagnostic substitution, changes in the law and other variables can result in a diagnosis being made more frequently, Diagnostic expansion occurs when loosened diagnostic criteria become widely accepted. Diagnostic substitution occurs when a diagnostic term is used in place of the label which had traditionally been attached to a category of patients. The law becomes a factor when it provides for services to patients with a particular diagnosis. Some physicians try to help their patients by using that diagnosis rather than an alternative which does not qualify them for assistance.[24]

REFERENCES

1. McNamara PH, Williams J, McCabe DJH, Walsh RA. Striking central pontine myelinolysis in a patient with alcohol dependence syndrome without hyponatremia. *JAMA Neurol.* 2016;73(2):234–235.

2. Wilbourn AJ. Value, limitations and pitfalls: false positive, false negative and indeterminate studies. In: *AAEE Course D: Radiculopathies.* Rochester, MN: American Association of Electromyography and Electrodiagnosis; 1989: 35–42.

3. Waldman W, Laureno R. Precautions for lumbar puncture: a survey of neurologic educators. *Neurology.* 1999;52(6):1296.

4. Jones T. Diagnosis of rheumatic fever. *JAMA.* 1944;126(8):481–484.

5. Special Writing Group. Guidelines for the diagnosis of rheumatic fever. Jones Criteria, 1992 update. Special Writing Group of the Committee on Rheumatic Fever, Endocarditis, and Kawasaki Disease of the Council on Cardiovascular Disease in the Young of the American Heart Association. *JAMA.* 1992;268(15):2069–2073.

6. Curatolo P, Moavero R, de Vries PJ. Neurological and neuropsychiatric aspects of tuberous sclerosis complex. *Lancet Neurol.* 2015;14(7):733–745.

7. Morris JC. Revised criteria for mild cognitive impairment may compromise the diagnosis of Alzheimer disease dementia. *Arch Neurol.* 2012;69(6):700–708.

8. Tuchman R, Rapin I. *Autism: a neurological disorder of early brain development.* London: MacKeith Press; 2006.

9. Mathew R, Bak TH, Hodges JR. Diagnostic criteria for corticobasal syndrome: a comparative study. *J Neurol Neurosurg Psychiatry*. 2012;83(4):405–410.

10. Lloyd TE, Mammen AL, Greenberg SA. Evolution and construction of diagnostic criteria for inclusion body myositis. Neurology. 2014;83:426–433.

11. Lee S, Chen C, Cugati S. Temporal arteritis. *Neurol Pract*. 2014;4(2):106–113.

12. Feldman HM, Reiff MI. Clinical practice. Attention deficit-hyperactivity disorder in children and adolescents. *N Engl J Med*. 2014;370(9):838–846

13. Saul R. *ADHD does not exist: the truth about attention deficit and hyperactivity disorder*. New York: Harper Collins; 2015.

14. Hinshaw SP, Scheffler RM. *The ADHD explosion: myths, medication, money, and today's push for performance*. New York: Oxford University Press; 2014.

15. Mestre TA, Gupta A, Lang AE. MRI signs of multiple system atrophy preceding the clinical diagnosis: the case for an imaging-supported probable MSA diagnostic category. *J Neurol Neurosurg Psychiatry*. 2016;87(4):443–444.

16. Pal G, Lin MM, Laureno R. Asterixis: a study of 103 patients. *Metab Brain Dis*. 2014;29(3):813–824.

17. Davis LE. Treachery of the hysterical diagnosis. *West J Med*. 1994;16(4):431.

18. Daum C, Hubschmid M, Aybek S. The value of "positive" clinical signs for weakness, sensory and gait disorders in conversion disorder: a systematic and narrative review. *J Neurol Neurosurg Psychiatry*. 2014;85(2):180–190.

19. Hurst JW. The value of using the entire New York Heart Association's classification of heart and vascular disease. *Clin Cardiol*. 2006;29(9):415–417.

20. Lüders H, Najm I, Wyllie E. Reply to "Of cabbages and kings: some considerations on classifications, diagnostic schemes, semiology, and concepts." *Epilepsia*. 2003;44(1):6–7.

21. Conomy J, Laureno R, Massariveh W. Transient behavioral syndrome associated with reversible vascular lesions of the fusiform-calcarine regions in humans. *Ann Neurol*. 1982;12(1):83.

22. Sha SJ, Layzer RB. Myasthenia gravis and Lambert-Eaton myasthenic syndrome in the same patient. *Muscle Nerve*. 2007;36(1):115–117.

23. Garvey M, and Laureno R. Hydrocephalus:obliterated perimesencephalic cisterns and the danger of sudden death. *Can J Neurol Sci*. 1998;25:154–158.

24. DeGraf WD, Miller G, Epstein LG, Rapin I. The autism "epidemic". *Neurology*. 2017;88:1371–1380.

4

Treatment

Our two goals are treatment of the disease and treatment of the patient. When considering a therapy, we weigh the benefits, the risks (Figures 4.1 and 4.2), and the costs; we consider patient-specific information; and we exercise judgment. Whenever possible, we provide reassurance, and we offer hope.

The practice of medicine is fundamentally an empirical process. For thousands of years, people have tried remedies. If one seemed to work, they continued to use it. If a method caused obvious harm, it was abandoned. This trial-and-error approach continues in modern medicine. There is scientific evidence for the utility of many medications for migraine. For a given patient, however, we proceed with a trial-and-error approach until we find one that is satisfactory. When phenytoin was first tried for treating epilepsy, its benefit was obvious. Perfect study design and statistics were not needed to "prove" its efficacy for human patients. In fact, Ernest Rutherford said that when a study needed statistics, the scientist should have done a better experiment.[1] We might say that when a therapy needs statistics, we should be looking for a better therapy.

Nevertheless, prospective, randomized, controlled studies do help us. Results are considered relevant when they are "statistically significant." We must remember that statistical significance was arbitrarily defined. When the chance is 1/20 or less that a finding could have occurred randomly, the result is considered "significant." There are limitations to this approach. First, a study of a therapy can show a "significantly positive" result by chance alone. Second, no clinician would disregard the dramatic therapeutic benefit of a treatment because the small number of patients in the study would mathematically allow for a 1/10 chance that benefit could have occurred by chance. He knows that the absence of statistical significance tells us nothing about the magnitude of

(A)

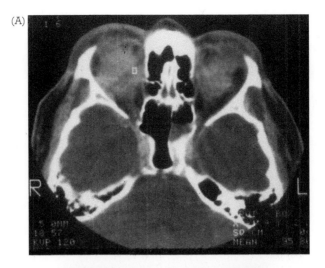

(B)

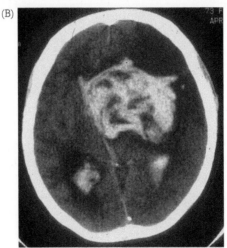

Figure 4.1 Examples of adverse effects of therapy. (A) Bilateral hemorrhage into the orbits in this patient, who had received heparin as part of the management of his finger injury. (B) This patient with atrial fibrillation had a large left middle cerebral artery distribution infarction. He received heparin immediately after his computed tomography (CT) scan was found to be normal. When he rapidly became obtunded, the repeat scan showed hemorrhagic transformation.

the impact a therapy can have. On a similar note, Ziliak and McClosky point out that some people imply that:

The value of a lottery ticket is the chance itself, the chance 1 in 38,000, say, or 1 in 100,000,000. It supposes that the only source of value in the lottery is

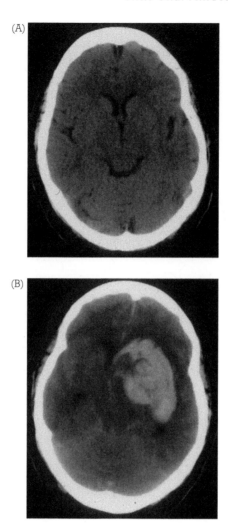

Figure 4.2 Adverse effect of therapy. The baseline (A) scan of a patient with an acute cerebral infarction and a repeat scan (B) following treatment with tissue plasminogen activator.

sampling variability. It sets aside as irrelevant—simply ignores—the value of the expected prize, the millions that success in the lottery could in fact yield. Setting aside both old and new criticisms of expected utility theory, a prize of $3.56 is very different, other things equal, from a prize of $356,000,000. No matter. Statistical significance, startlingly, ignores the difference.[2]

Ziliak and McCloskey give a medical example. For helping Mother to lose weight, one considers:

Two diet pills with identical prices and side effects. You are determined to choose one of the two pills for her.

The first pill, named Oomph, will on average take off twenty pounds. But it is very uncertain in its effects—at plus or minus ten pounds (you can if you wish take "plus or minus" here to signify technically "two standard errors around the mean"). Oomph gives a big effect, you see but with a high variance.

Alternatively the pill Precision will take off five pounds on average. But it is much more certain in its effects. Choosing Precision entails a probable error of plus or minus a mere one-half pound. Pill Precision is estimated, in other words, much more precisely than is Oomph, at any rate in view of the sampling schemes that measured the amount of variation in each.

So which pill for Mother, whose goal is to lose weight?

The problem we are describing is that the sizeless sciences—from agronomy to zoology—choose Precision over Oomph every time . . .

But Precision is obviously the wrong choice. Wrong for Mother's weight management program and wrong for the many other victims of the sizeless scientist. The sizeless scientist decides whether something is important or not—she decides "whether there exists an effect," as she puts it—by looking not at the something's oomph but at how precisely it is estimated. Diet pill Oomph is potent, she admits. But, after all, it is very imprecise, promising to shed anything from 10 to 30 pounds. Diet pill Precision will, by contrast, shed only 4.5 to 5.5 pounds, she concedes, but, goodness, it is very precise—in Fisher's terms, very statistically significant.[2]

Shorvon and colleagues have emphasized that "evidence-based medicine," with its rigorous reviews of the methodology of medical articles, does not help the neurologist when the existing evidence does not meet the high standards required.[3] Often scientific analysis reveals imperfections of the evidence for a treatment benefit or adverse effect. However, the inadequacy of evidence does not relieve the neurologist of his or her responsibility to educate and treat the patient. His decisions are based on the best evidence available, including systematic reviews of evidence and therapeutic guidelines written by groups of experts.

Because of the lack of good evidence, systematic reviews often result in recommendations that are "tentative and largely already well-known." [3] Systematic reviews are very helpful when a disease, like Bell's palsy, tends to improve without treatment. In these disorders, a great variety of treatments can be suspected to be helpful. When the data are poor, a systematic review can yield strong conclusions. The Cochrane Library, as of 2012, could state that in Bell's palsy the evidence for benefit of hyperbaric oxygen is very low in

quality and that the evidence for acupuncture is inadequate. Such strong negative statements are very helpful to the clinician.

When, in spite of systematic review, the utility of a treatment is uncertain,
therapeutic guidelines can be helpful. Typically, a group of experts, often
under the aegis of a medical society or association, will propound guidelines
for therapy. The Neurocritical Care Society published guidelines for the management of status epilepticus. (SE) "Due to the paucity of controlled clinical
trial data regarding the treatment of SE, the writing committee of SE experts
surveyed a select group of international SE experts."[4]

Evidence does not always trump such consensus opinion. For example,
one may have diligently reviewed all articles gleaned by using relevant search
terms. Sometimes an article found by using the search terms does not use
appropriate criteria for the diagnosis of the disorder in question. The review,
however, may not take this deficiency into account.[5] In such a situation, a consensus guideline might be better than a systematic literature review.

Standardized evidence-based protocols are sometimes formalized as algo-
rithms. They are typically displayed as decision trees. Such a structured approach
can be beneficial for students, young doctors, and nonphysician clinicians.
A drawback is the potential for unnecessary rigidity. An algorithm designed
by a consensus panel may recommend one drug family for the initial treatment
of a disease. However, an experienced neurologist may prefer another type of
medication for a given patient. In the era of the electronic medical record, deviation from an algorithm may be perceived as a "quality" problem, especially if
there is an adverse effect of the medication chosen.

EARLY TREATMENT

For fulminant vasculitis or bacterial meningitis, starting treatment sooner is
clearly better than starting treatment later. When a treatment has been shown
to work for a less florid disease, experts speculate that it would work better had
it been started earlier. The urge to treat early is so strong that authorities sometimes gradually loosen diagnostic criteria for a disease in order to allow earlier
treatment.[6] Of course, loosening of diagnostic criteria and treatment before a
diagnosis is clear means that more people will receive therapy for a disease that
they do not have. Nevertheless, if the treatment is relatively benign, it maybe
reasonable to treat for a presumptive diagnosis.

The idea that early treatment is good can become the last refuge of a com-
mitted doctor. Long after surgery had been abandoned for Bell's palsy, I was
told by a neuro-otologist that the surgery is effective, that the problem with
outcomes was that the operation is not done soon enough. As the era of

anticoagulation for acute stroke was waning, a stroke specialist informed me that anticoagulation was effective, that the key was to start it early enough. True believers are not always wrong, but they must generate data to convert us to using their therapies.

THERAPEUTIC EXPANSION

There are various ways that clinicians try to expand their armamentarium. When a mode of therapy seems useful for one disorder, some doctors will try that treatment for another condition. If a therapy based on a certain rationale seems useful, a doctor will try other treatments based on the same rationale as the first. When there is an association of two conditions, a doctor will, sooner or later, try to treat one disorder by treating the other. These therapeutic forays can lead to important advances as well as misadventures.

Broadened use is often seen with anticonvulsant medicines. After phenytoin was found to be useful for treating epilepsy, it was tried for many other diseases.[7] Levetiracetam was proved useful for adjunctive treatment of epilepsy. Soon thereafter, doctors tried it as monotherapy. When medications (e.g., valproic acid) were proved effective for treating patients with seizures, many were utilized for therapy of mood disorders.

In metastatic malignancies, benefit was found from treatment with a monoclonal antibody targeting vascular endothelial growth factor. Subsequently, doctors used the same antibody to treat radiation necrosis of the spinal cord in cancer patients. In this latter instance, there was no clear rationale for such broadened use. It seems that some doctors, once they are familiar with using a treatment for one disease, are willing to try that therapy for another.

Broadened use occurs not only with medications but also with devices. By the time a study showing the benefit of an older stent retriever has been published,[8] a new stent retriever may have been invented. Based on their experience, some doctors may prefer the new device to the proven one. They assume that the data about the older device are relevant to the new device, for which the rationale is the same. Other doctors may insist that a study be done to show equivalent benefit with the new device.

Once a new therapeutic approach has proved effective in treating one disease, doctors try using it for other conditions. After a guinea pig serum was a success in treating diphtheria, physicians produced another antitoxin for treatment of tetanus. After successes with serum treatment of bacterial toxic diseases, a horse serum was tried less successfully to treat a viral disease, poliomyelitis. Providing passive immunity continues to be an important method of treatment for botulism and other diseases.

When two disorders are found to be associated, the idea occurs that one condition may cause or influence the other. The occasional occurrence of thymoma in myasthenia gravis was noted. Some patients seemed to do well after the thymomas were removed. As a result, doctors decided to try removing nontumorous thymus glands from myasthenia gravis patients. They had the impression that the patients benefitted. This surgery continued to be performed for 75 years in spite of it never having been subjected to a double-blind, randomized, controlled prospective study.[9]

Although thymectomy had never been proved to benefit myasthenia gravis, there was much disagreement over those 75 years about how to do thymectomy. Some felt that it was important to open the chest, thereby allowing the surgeon to inspect the anterior mediastinum and remove every bit of thymus. Others preferred a less invasive trans-sternal method that allows good visualization of most of the thymus. Still others preferred a transcervical approach that is even less invasive and still allows removal of much of the thymus. There had been more discussion of different surgical methods than there had been effort to determine whether thymectomy is truly effective. As of 2013, the Cochrane Library found that a randomized controlled study is necessary to determine whether thymectomy is useful. Finally, in 2016, there was published support for the surgery. The study was randomized and controlled but neither treating doctors nor patients were blinded.[10]

In diseases other than myasthenia gravis, we see the same problem: academic contention about which treatment is best when neither has been proved. We see other behaviors, which are hopeful but not based on evidence. We see sequential use of modestly beneficial treatments for a disease when there is no proof of an additive benefit. We even see discussion about what sequence of treatments to use for a disease when the disease itself is ill-defined.

Decisions about treatment must take into account all information available about the clinical situation. At a particular time, animal data, biochemical knowledge, case series reports, and personal experience may be critical to management decisions. Certainly, these types of information are important when there is no "proper" controlled study. Even when there is a controlled study, it may not be directly applicable to a specific patient, and the physician must rely on well-focused case series evidence.

Unfortunately, the urge to treat can trump the evidence. When a disease is known to commonly have a disastrous outcome, the neurologist is inclined to prescribe. "You have to try something" is the thought process. Hence, heparin was given for basilar artery thrombosis for many decades before being abandoned. Cyclophosphamide was given for decades to treat patients with aggressive multiple sclerosis without good evidence for benefit. Due to concern that a berry aneurysm might bleed again, neurosurgeons used to clamp carotid arteries. As one would expect, therapeutic occlusion of a carotid artery did not always end well.

The medical community makes great effort to be scientific. Nevertheless, when the data are not clear, one's assessment of the risks and benefits can be swayed by therapeutic trends. Sometimes, as Maurice Victor put it, treatment preference "depends on which way the pack is running" (Maurice Victor, MD, in conversation, 1974).

PRESUMPTIVE DIAGNOSIS

There are circumstances when it is best to proceed with treatment although the diagnosis is uncertain. "The greater the relative benefit of therapy, the less certain physicians need to be before initiating empirical therapy; the greater the relative risk of therapy, the more certain they must be."[11] Depression is a prime example. With depression the stakes are high: a patient may suffer without treatment. The risk of medication is not great compared to the potential benefit in this situation. When in doubt about the diagnosis, it is best to treat. The response to medication may clarify the diagnosis.

Sometimes the situation will guide the neurologist's decision to treat. A patient who long ago underwent bariatric surgery may report dizziness for which there is no clear explanation. The neurologist suspects vitamin deficiency. He searches for signs of Wernicke disease and carefully documents normal cognitive function, extraocular movements, coordination, and tandem gait. The brain imaging is normal. Although he cannot diagnose Wernicke disease, he should treat for it. The context of a bariatric surgery patient who takes no vitamins dictates treatment without diagnosis. The treatment, thiamine, is relatively safe. If there is, in fact, smoldering Wernicke disease, the gain of treatment is great.

Herpes simplex encephalitis is another disease for which treatment should be initiated when the disease is suspected, not proved. For years, some authorities advocated a definite diagnosis by brain biopsy before treating herpes simplex encephalitis. Because misdiagnosis was not rare and because vidarabine was a toxic medication, the case for biopsy was strong. Three changes occurred. First, acyclovir was found to be a safer and more effective treatment than vidarabine. Second, herpes simplex–specific polymerase chain reaction (PCR) was developed as a very sensitive and specific test for viral DNA in the spinal fluid. Third, magnetic resonance imaging (MRI) became widely available. The availability of benign tests and a safe medicine weakened the case for brain biopsy. When one suspects that a patient has herpes encephalitis, he should begin treatment while awaiting the PCR result.

PATIENT EDUCATION

Setting appropriate expectations is important. Giving a medicine to help the pain of diabetic neuropathy, I typically explain that we are trying to alleviate, not eliminate, the pain and that we cannot change the numbness due to neuropathy. Raymond De Paulo tells a patient that the ultimate goal is to make his depression 80% better 80% of the time (personal communication in conversation, 1993). No improvement can be expected from treatment of multiple sclerosis, one must tell the patient. The goal of therapy is to lessen future clinical episodes and accumulation of brain lesions. Repetition of the goals and expectations is important. Many patients, hoping for a cure, do not absorb or remember what the doctor says about the limited goals of a therapy. One teaching session is often not enough.

Successful treatment of a chronic neurologic problem only comes by developing a long-term relationship with a patient. Explaining the therapeutic process to patients is critical to success. For migraine and epilepsy, the patient should understand the trial-and-error nature of the treatment process. He must know that, for a particular person, one dose may be effective, but for another a higher dose may be needed. For one patient, a single medication may be adequate, but for another more than one will be necessary. Patients are more likely to maintain a relationship with a doctor when they understand that they are entering into a scientifically guided trial-and-error process, that there may not be instant success. With this understanding, they are less likely to give up on the doctor when the initial prescription is unsuccessful.

EASE OF USE

Patients and doctors prefer medications that are easy to use. Patients find that taking a medicine once a day is easy. Doctors like medication regimens with which patients are more likely to comply. Levetiracetam is an example. A twice-daily regimen was approved for use as adjunctive therapy for epilepsy. Everybody liked the idea that it was useful when taken only twice a day. When neurologists began to use it as monotherapy, they were wise if they attended to the medicine's basic pharmacology: it is a short half-life medicine. It is often more effective as monotherapy when given 3 or 4 times daily, in spite of its being approved and advertised as a twice-daily drug. Both ease of use and efficacy are not always achievable.

In Parkinson disease patients, we try to minimize complications of therapy with L-dopa/carbidopa or dopaminergic agents. We explain, at the beginning of the relationship, that small frequent doses of the medicine are less likely to cause dyskinesia and other complications than are larger, less frequent doses.

Many patients, with this initial education, are willing to comply with the inconvenience of frequent doses.

NONCOMPLIANCE

Nonadherence to therapy wastes resources. The common example is the epileptic who does not take his medicine, resulting in repeated admissions to the hospital for convulsions. In the absence of confusion or dementia, noncompliance is due to a wide range of psychiatric disorders. How one can get certain alcoholic patients to conscientiously take antiseizure medication, I have not learned. In a person with an affective disorder, appropriate antidepressant medication can sometimes change the patient's attitude and facilitate compliance.

NEUROSURGERY

When there is uncertainty about the proper treatment, we must inform the patient. Should one recommend radiosurgery for an acoustic neuroma while it is small because the surgery will be more dangerous when the tumor has enlarged? Should surgery be done on a very large acoustic neuroma that is compressing the brainstem, or should one, at that point, be content with a ventricular shunt for hydrocephalus? Patient age, patient risk averseness, and the experience of the surgeon all play into decision-making. It is often helpful to show a patient images of the tumor so that he can better appreciate his situation. Ultimately, however, the neurologist's recommendation depends on his judgment about the case. Often the opinion of a neurosurgeon is needed.

When the neurologist refers a patient to a surgeon, he can lose control of case management. Many times, I have explained to a patient that his problem is not an emergency. "We will get the opinion of a surgeon. Should the surgeon suggest an operation, I want you to come back to discuss his recommendation with me." Too often, I next hear about the patient when I receive the operative report. Somehow, when the surgeon tells the patient that he needs an operation, the patient receives the statement as definitive. Many patients need clarity and fear ambiguity. It is always a challenge to get the patient to revisit, to discuss his options before he undergoes surgery.

The inpatient is at a great disadvantage in "negotiating" with the surgeon. Half naked and supine in a hospital bed, a patient is not in the best position to discuss his options. Thus, for elective surgery, I avoid the convenience of having the surgeon see the patient while he is still in the hospital. It is often better for the patient, rested and dressed, to sit across from the surgeon in the outpatient department.

REASSURANCE

Reassurance is an important aspect of therapeutics. Reassurance does not mean telling a patient, "Don't worry about it." On the contrary, Maurice Victor taught residents to never utter these words. To emphasize the point, he would say to residents, "You will have to repeat a year of residency. It's okay—don't worry about it."

It is not possible to reassure a patient without spending time. The patient must feel that he has been carefully evaluated. Without his perceiving that he is in the hands of a careful doctor, he cannot feel reassured.

Skill at reassurance can, to some extent, be learned. The technique is to offer encouragement rather than to emphasize disease. Take, for example, a patient blinded in one eye by an optic neuropathy. When no recovery is evident over a period of months, a good approach is to emphasize the positive. Kessel relates the story of a doctor who spent a long time examining a good eye, telling the patient how perfect it was and how fortunate he was to have such an eye, "good enough to do the work of two without any difficulty."[12]

"The reassuring doctor must appear strong, reassuring, firm in his purpose, absolutely dependable, unable to be upset by anything the patient may say or do, unflustered, unembarrassable, unassailable, and free from weakness."[12] Few of us can achieve this level of perfection, but many can learn to have the appearance, to practice behaviors that reassure patients and families. As a young neurologist, I would be upset and anxious as I went to meet with families of patients who had remained comatose after surviving cardiac arrest. I was sad for the patients and families. Then, one day, I read about a local congresswoman who had been in a vegetative state for several months following a cardiac arrest. In a newspaper article about her predicament, the patient's daughter was quoted as saying, "I haven't met a smiling neurologist yet." I suddenly realized that smiling might not be inappropriate. The relatives already knew that the situation was grave; they did not need another somber presence. I began to abandon a serious face and to force myself to gently smile as I approached these families. As a result, they usually perceived me as confident and competent. For a year or more, I had to act to make myself smile until one day I realized that smiling in such situations had become natural, a habit really.

The neurologist should make time to think before speaking. Zinsser recalled the advice he had received: "Act thoughtful; and if you don't know what to say, say nothing; but say nothing deliberately and slowly."[13] Kessel recalled being advised to take as long as necessary to wash his hands in order to have time to think about what he would tell the patient at the end of a consultation.[12]

In the most severe and clear-cut cases of brain disease, the family must be told the dismal truth and be helped to face reality. However, except in the most advanced cases, the neurologist must not extinguish hope. To a family whose child had a deep-seated malignant glioma, Wilder Penfield would say, "I am afraid your little boy is going to die. But I may be wrong. Doctors are wrong sometimes, you know."[14] As long as the door is not quite shut, families and patients draw succor from a glimmer of hope.

According to Kessel, the deepest level of reassurance comes when the doctor tells the patient that no matter what he may have to go through in his illness, he will be able to bear it "with my help."[12] The comforting message is that, "the patient will not be abandoned."

In sum, neurologic treatment involves the provision of hope and reassurance. Of course, it requires pharmacologic surgical and physical therapies. It also requires the good judgment to withhold therapies when it is in the patient's best interest. Robert Hutchison proposed a physician's prayer: "From inability to let well enough alone; from too much zeal for the new and contempt for what is old; from putting knowledge before wisdom, science before art, and cleverness before common sense, from treating patients as cases, and from making the cure of the disease more grievous than endurance of the same, Good Lord, deliver us."[15]

REFERENCES

1. Kassirer JP. Clinical trials and meta-analysis. What do they do for us? *N Engl J Med.* 1992;327(4):273–274.
2. Ziliak S. *The cult of statistical significance: how the standard error costs us jobs, justice, and lives.* Ann Arbor: University of Michigan Press; 2011.
3. Shorvon SD, Tomson T, Cock HR. The management of epilepsy during pregnancy—progress is painfully slow. *Epilepsia.* 2009;50(5):973–974.
4. Brophy GM, Bell R, Claassen J, Alldredge B, Bleck TP, Glaser T, Larouche S, et al. Guidelines for the evaluation and management of status epilepticus. *Neurocrit Care.* 2012;17(1):3–23.
5. Halperin JJ, Kurlan R, Schwalb JM, Cusimano MD, Gronseth G, Gloss D. Practice guideline: idiopathic normal pressure hydrocephalus: Response to shunting and predictors of response: Report of the Guideline Development, Dissemination, and Implementation Subcommittee of the American Academy of Neurology. *Neurology.* 2015;85(23):2063–2071.
6. Miller AE and Pelletier. Multiple sclerosis: rapid diagnosis or right diagnosis. *Neurology.* 2016;87:652–653.
7. Dreyfus J. *The story of a remarkable medicine.* Herndon, VA: Lentern Books; 2002.

8. Touma L, Filion KB, Sterling LH, Atallah R, Windle SB, Eisenberg MJ. Stent retrievers for the treatment of acute ischemic stroke: a systematic review and meta-analysis of randomized clinical trials. *JAMA Neurol.* 2016;73(3):275–281.

9. Gronseth GS, Barohn RJ. Practice parameter: thymectomy for autoimmune myasthenia gravis (an evidence-based review): report of the Quality Standards Subcommittee of the American Academy of Neurology. *Neurology.* 2000;55(1):7–15.

10. Wolfe GI, Kaminski HJ, Aban IB, Minisman G, Kuo HC, Marx A, Ströbel P, et al. Randomized trial of thymectomy in myasthenia gravis. *N Engl J Med.* 2016;375(6):511–522.

11. Pauker SG, Kopelman RI. How sure is sure enough? *N Engl J Med.* 1992;326(10):688–691.

12. Kessel N. Reassurance. *Lancet.* 1979;313(8126):1128–1133.

13. Zinsser H. *As I remember him: the biography of R. S.* Boston, MA: Little Brown and Company; 1940.

14. Penfield W. *No man alone: a neurosurgeon's life.* Boston, MA: Little Brown and Company; 1977.

15. Hutchison R. Modern treatment. *Br Med J.* 1953;1(4811):671.

PART TWO

Topics in Neurologic Disease

5

Symmetry

Bilateral symmetry is the hallmark of chemically caused brain diseases. The pathology is more or less the same on the right and left sides of the brain, whether the cause is metabolic, nutritional, toxic, or hereditary (e.g., enzyme deficiency). Thus, bilateral symmetry is very important to the clinical neurologist. When brain images show symmetric brain lesions, the neurologist should think about which chemical disorder could be the cause. When there is no evident explanation for symmetric lesions, the symmetry may be an important clue to a brain disease of unknown cause, such as a toxin.

Symmetry is not limited to diseases that are chemically based. Symmetry is common in the pathology of degenerative diseases. Furthermore, symmetry can occur in cerebrovascular disease, infection, trauma, and other disease families. In fact, symmetry is not limited to disease of the central nervous system. For mechanical reasons, symmetrical mononeuropathies can occur.

CHEMICAL/METABOLIC DISEASE

Chemical and metabolic encephalopathies can be caused by problems with substrate (glucose and oxygen), derangements of electrolytes, organ failure, endocrine dysfunction, nutritional deficiency, exogenous toxins, and hereditary enzyme deficiencies. When fixed brain injury occurs, the damage is more or less symmetric. Hypoxic-ischemic encephalopathies affect the brain symmetrically (Figure 5.1). In cardiac arrest, for example, the patient must survive long enough for lesions to become visible. Hypoglycemic brain damage is similar. Vitamin deficiencies can cause symmetric lesions. In Wernicke disease, the symmetric lesions are mainly in the periventricular gray matter around

(A)

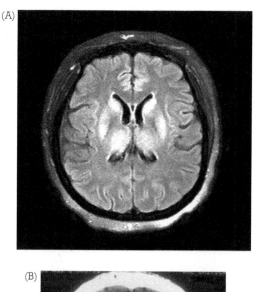

(B)

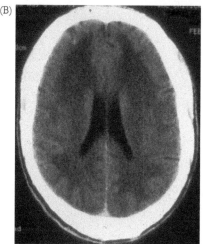

Figure 5.1 Two examples of symmetric brain damage after cardiac arrest. (A) Acute striatal and thalamic lesions. (B) Symmetry in delayed post-anoxic demyelination.

the third and fourth ventricles. Vitamin B_{12} deficiency, on the other hand, primarily affects white matter in the spinal cord. In organ failure, it is liver disease that best illustrates symmetry. Acute liver failure can cause reversible increased magnetic resonance imaging (MRI) signal intensity in the globus pallidus and other structures and regions. In patients with repeated episodes of hepatic coma, fixed, symmetric lesions can develop. Hereditary forms of metabolic disease also cause symmetric brain lesions. In hereditary hepatocerebral disease (Wilson disease), for example, there is symmetrically altered MRI signal in the thalamus, midbrain tegmentum, caudate, putamen, and globus pallidus. Hereditary leukodystrophies produce symmetric areas of altered signal in the cerebral white matter. The typical lesion distribution varies from one leukodystrophy to another but is not absolutely specific. Hereditary metabolic diseases of gray matter like citrullinemia cause symmetric abnormality of the cerebral cortex.

Exogenous chemicals that affect the brain do so symmetrically. There are many examples. Methanol poisoning survivors develop symmetric brain and optic nerve lesions. Patients who have inadvertently inhaled dichloroacetylene (a trichloroethylene break down product) develop bilateral trigeminal neuropathies. Ingestion of mold, which has developed on improperly stored grain, can cause symmetric brain lesions. In these cases, the mycotoxin, 3-nitropropionic acid, is responsible for bilateral striatal injury. Residual thiocyanate in inadequately processed cassava root (a dietary staple in some regions) can cause bilateral leukoencephalopathy (Figure 5.2). "Recreational" drug use such as "ecstasy," an amphetamine derivative, can also cause symmetric toxic leukoencephalopathy. Medications can likewise cause symmetric brain changes. The antiseizure medication vigabatrin can cause symmetric reversible MRI hyperintensity in thalamus, midbrain tectum, globus pallidus, and cerebellar white matter. Metronidazole, the antiparasitic medicine, can cause symmetric abnormal MRI signal in the dentate nuclei. These are only a few examples.

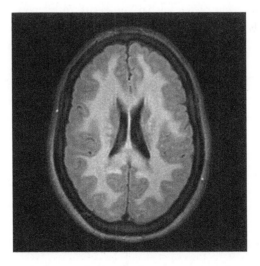

Figure 5.2 Symmetric leukoencephalopathy due to ingestion of cassava root.

VASCULAR DISEASE

When symmetric lesions develop in vascular disease of brain, the underlying anatomy is responsible. This statement holds true for borderzone, occlusive arterial, veno-occlusive and aneurysmal disease. For example, the anterior spinal artery, single and midline, supplies the ventral spinal cord symmetrically. When it is occluded, the resulting infarction is bilateral and symmetric.

The symmetry in border zone ischemia occurs when the distribution of the major arteries is similar on the right and left sides of the brain. With hypotension, there can result symmetric infarction in the border zones. Typically, these occur between the anterior cerebral artery (ACA) and middle cerebral artery (MCA) territories. Similarly, there can occur symmetric border zone infarcts between the MCA and posterior cerebral artery (PCA) territories (Figure 5.3A). There can be bilateral occipital infarcts at the border zone of the supply of all three major cerebral arteries: the MCA, ACA, and PCA. The cerebellum can show symmetric border zone infarcts between the posterior inferior cerebellar and superior cerebellar artery territories (SCA) (Figure 5.3B).

Depending on the underlying anatomy, interesting symmetric infarctions may occur. For example, bilateral middle cerebellar peduncle (MCP) infarcts can occur with bilateral vertebral artery occlusion. This pattern of symmetric anterior inferior cerebellar artery (AICA) infarction has been explained by the MCP being in the border zone of the AICA and the SCA in some patients(Figure 5.4A).[1] Since both PCAs originate from the basilar artery, a single embolus to the top of the basilar can result in bilateral PCA distribution infarction(Figure 5.4B). Usually, perforating arteries arise from the proximal portions of the PCAs. Occasionally, however, there is a unilateral thalamoperforating artery which then bifurcates into two branches, one going to the right and one to the left thalamus. If this artery of Percheron becomes occluded, symmetric thalamic infarctions occur (Figure 5.5A). If the proximal (A1) segment of the ACA is congenitally absent, the one ACA supplies the ACA territory bilaterally. Occlusion of that vessel can result in bilaterally symmetric infarctions (Figure 5.5B).

Venous as well as arterial disease can cause symmetric brain findings. The superior sagittal sinus is single and midline; its occlusion can result in bihemispheric infarction. Also single and midline is the straight sinus, whose occlusion can cause bithalamic infarction (Figure 5.6A). Likewise midline is the superior vermian vein, occlusion of which can cause bilateral infarction of the cerebellum.

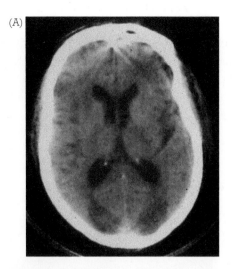

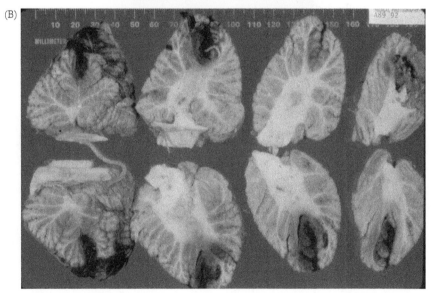

Figure 5.3 Symmetric infarctions in border zones imply a symmetric underlying arterial supply. (A) Posterior cerebral–middle cerebral artery border zone infarcts. (B) Symmetric hemorrhagic infarcts in the superior cerebellar–posterior inferior cerebellar artery border zones.

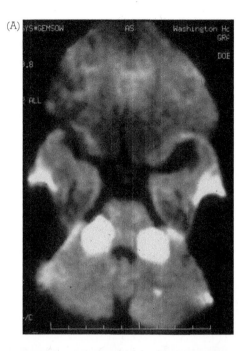

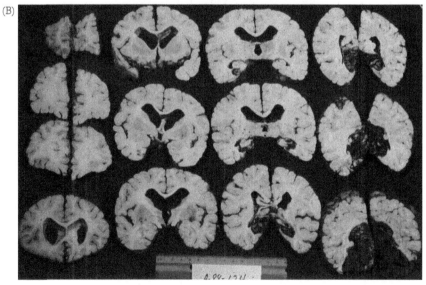

Figure 5.4 Symmetric infarctions. (A) Bilateral infarction of the middle cerebellar peduncle, which has been considered a border zone in some patients. (B) Symmetric hemorrhagic infarctions in the posterior cerebral artery distribution. The usual cause is embolism to the top of the basilar artery, which typically gives rise to both posterior cerebral arteries.

(A)

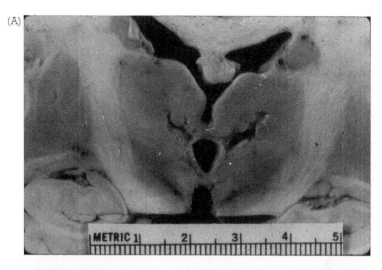

(B)

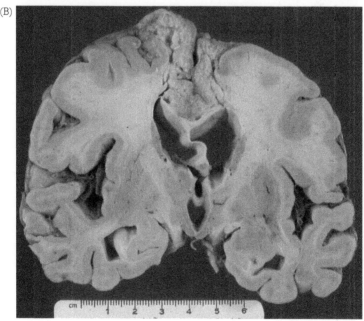

Figure 5.5 Symmetric infarctions. (A) Bilateral thalamic infarctions typically due to occlusion of the artery of Percheron. (B) Bilateral anterior cerebral artery distribution infarction can occur when a single ACA supplies the right and left sides.

Because an anterior communicating artery aneurysm is midline, its rupture can cause symmetric hemorrhage in the frontal lobes. The hematomas can be continuous across the genu and anterior body of the corpus callosum.

Finally, small-vessel vasculitis can occasionally present with symmetric brain lesions (Figure 5.6B).

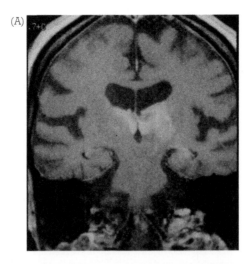

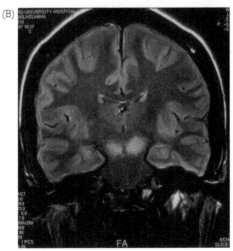

Figure 5.6 Symmetric lesions in vascular disease. (A) Venous infarctions of the thalami due to straight sinus occlusion. (B) Symmetric lesions due to pathologically proven small-vessel vasculitis.

NEOPLASTIC DISEASE

Although symmetry is not typical in neoplastic disease, it is not unknown. Symmetry, when present, is often due to midline anatomical features. The falx cerebri is midline. If the patient develops a meningioma of this structure, it can grow to the right and left, creating a "dumbbell meningioma." The corpus callosum is a central single structure. When a glioma develops there, it can spread bilaterally to form a "butterfly glioma." Lymphoma in the corpus callosum can also spread both ways (Figure 5.7A). Glioma and primary central nervous system (CNS) lymphoma can also occur symmetrically, independent of a midline connection. Two examples are bilateral thalamic glioma and bilateral periventricular lymphoma. Beautifully symmetric cerebellar lymphoma has been reported. Clearly, a genetic predisposition is present when symmetric jugular paragangliomas occur or when symmetric eighth-nerve schwannomas develop in neurofibromatosis type 2. Even in metastatic disease one may see remarkable symmetry. If carcinoma metastasizes to one cavernous sinus, it

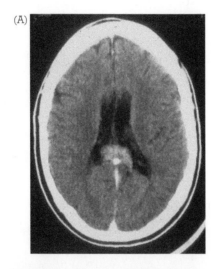

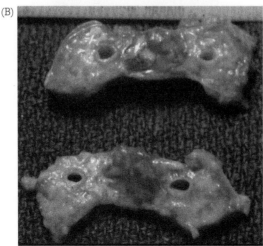

Figure 5.7 Symmetry in malignancy. (A) Lymphoma of the corpus callosum. (B) Metastatic cancer filling both cavernous sinuses. The pituitary gland is in the center of each coronal section.

may spread to the opposite sinus. Such bilateral cavernous sinus tumor can cause total paralysis of extraocular movement (Figure 5.7B).

INFECTIOUS DISEASE

Certain CNS infections can show bilateral symmetry (Figure 5.8). Poliomyelitis is an example. Inflammation and neuronal damage of the anterior horns of the spinal cord is often, but not always, symmetric. The anterior horn cells and

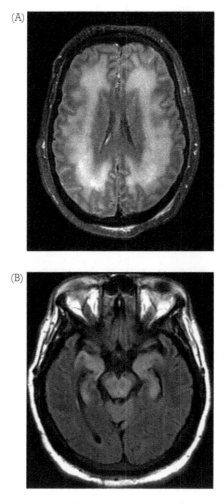

Figure 5.8 Symmetry in infectious disease. (A) Leukoencephalopathy in acute influenza. (B) Pathologically proven rabies encephalitis. (Provided by Mary Carter Denny, MD.)

certain brainstem nuclei are also selectively vulnerable to other enteroviruses. In recent decades, West Nile virus has come to the United States; this arbovirus can cause an identical symmetric syndrome. Regardless of the specific viral cause, an axial MRI scan can show remarkably symmetric anterior horn disease in a given case at a given spinal cord level. West Nile virus can also cause symmetric lesions of the thalamus, substantia nigra, and other structures. In the transmissible spongiform encephalopathies, there are characteristically symmetric hyperintense signal abnormalities on diffusion-weighted MRI images.

OTHER DISEASES

Symmetric lesions can appear in many categories of disease. For examples, closed head injury can cause symmetric brain contusions, and surgical intervention can leave symmetric lesions (Figure 5.9). In addition, the pathology of most of the degenerative diseases is more or less symmetric (Figure 5.10). Thus the spinal cord in Friedreich ataxia or the Wallerian degeneration of the corticospinal tract seen on images in primary lateral sclerosis are predictably symmetric. Demyelinative disease is classically multifocal rather than bilaterally symmetric. On occasion, however, acute disseminated encephalomyelitis or acute necrotizing hemorrhagic leukoencephalitis can cause remarkably symmetric lesions (Figure 5.11).

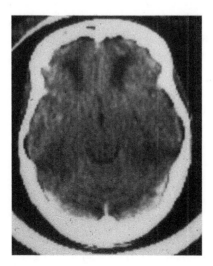

Figure 5.9 Symmetry from the intentional trauma of bifrontal leukotomy.

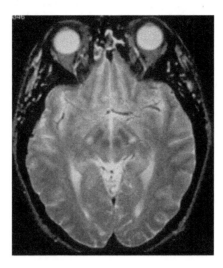

Figure 5.10 Symmetry in degenerative disease. The increased signal in the corticospinal tracts in the midbrain is due to primary lateral sclerosis.

PERIPHERAL NEUROLOGY

Well known is the symmetry that occurs in the polyneuropathies. Symmetric mononeuropathies (e.g., ascites compressing both lateral femoral cutaneous nerves) are not uncommon. A special type occurs when generalized acute muscle necrosis causes bilateral anterior compartment swelling, which in turn compresses the peroneal nerves. The resulting bilateral peroneal neuropathy can be transient or permanent. I have seen hypothyroid myopathy cause bilateral peroneal neuropathy. James Corbett has seen similar bilateral peroneal neuropathies result from the combination of intense exercise and hypokalemia in hyperaldosteronism (James J. Corbett, MD, in conversation c. 1995).

Special forms of trauma can result in symmetric peripheral nerve injuries. Anterior-posterior traumatic compression of the pelvis has caused symmetric severe femoral neuropathies. The patient in a reported case underwent such compression when he was caught in a machine.[2] I have observed severe bilateral femoral stretch neuropathy in an intoxicated man who fell asleep with his buttocks on a wooden bed frame; his legs hung forward as his upper body lay supine on the lower half of the mattress. Stupor also predisposed to paralysis in a heroin user. She sat on a hard floor, in the yoga lotus position, and injected herself. She was uncertain as to the duration of her narcosis in the seated position. Eventually she awakened

(A)

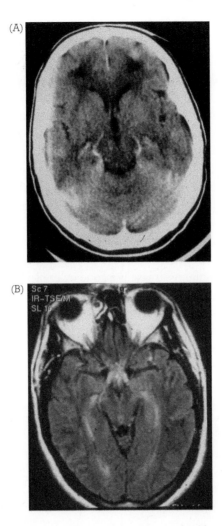

(B)

Figure 5.11 Symmetry in demyelinative disease. (A) Cerebral lesions of acute disseminated encephalomyelitis. (B) Multiple sclerosis affecting both optic tracts.

with profound bilateral sciatic neuropathy. I have also observed a burn victim who underwent general anesthesia for leg amputation: he awoke from surgery with bilateral hand and arm paralysis from right and left brachial plexus stretch injuries. In each of these cases, symmetric compression or stretch superimposed on symmetric normal anatomy resulted in disabling symmetric mononeuropathies.

FINAL COMMENTS

1. Symmetry can be a problem for the neurologist (Figure 5.12). Especially on computed tomography (CT) scans, symmetric disease can be difficult to notice on the background of symmetric brain anatomy. The eye more quickly detects a one-sided lesion or multifocal asymmetric lesions than symmetric lesions.
2. Symmetry of brain lesions is important to the clinician because it suggests a toxic, metabolic, or other chemically based cause. When central pontine myelinolysis was first described, for example, the symmetry of the disease suggested a metabolic cause. In due time, a metabolic cause was found.
3. Symmetry is helpful to the investigator. Diseases with symmetric pathology but unknown cause probably are chemically based. Marchiafava-Bignami disease is a good example. The clue of symmetry gives investigators an opportunity to pursue a metabolic or toxic cause. Likewise, symmetrical lesions in unnamed and unknown diseases should suggest a chemical cause like a toxin.

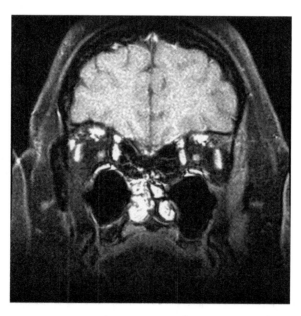

Figure 5.12 The symmetry of bilateral optic neuritis makes it difficult to notice the enhancement of the optic nerves unless the scan is carefully compared to the unenhanced scan.

REFERENCES

1. Akiyama K, Takizawa S, Tokuoka K, Ohnuki Y, Kobayashi N, Shinohara Y. Bilateral middle cerebellar peduncle infarction caused by traumatic vertebral artery dissection. *Neurology.* 2001;56(5):693–694.
2. D'Amelio LF, Musser DJ, Rhodes M. Bilateral femoral nerve neuropathy following blunt trauma. Case report. *J Neurosurg.* 1990;73(4):630–632.

6

Selective Vulnerability

In one disease, certain areas of brain are particularly vulnerable. In other diseases, different parts of the brain are more susceptible. This was the observation of Cècile and Oskar Vogt.[1] As a concept, *selective vulnerability* was readily accepted. Its basis in anoxic encephalopathy, however, gave rise to dispute. The Vogts' idea was that the neurons of the Sommer sector (CA1 region) of the hippocampus were by nature selectively predisposed to anoxic injury. Walter Spielmeyer, on the other hand, attributed the disproportionate anoxic damage of the Sommer sector to its poor arterial supply. The agreement of the prominent pathologists, however, is more important than their dispute. Regardless of mechanism, they accepted the notion of selective vulnerability in brain disease. The concept of selective vulnerability was originally applied to toxic/metabolic and hereditary disorders. It is also useful in thinking about other neuropathologic processes including neoplastic, infectious, demyelinative, vascular, and traumatic diseases.

TRAUMA

In closed-head trauma, which can do all sorts of damage to the nervous system, contusion is the best example of special vulnerability. When a solid surface stops the head's movement, the brain is whipped about.[2] In the process, it may slosh against the skull. Irrespective of the impact site, the frontal and temporal lobes of the brain are the areas most likely to be contused. Various theories have been proposed to explain this selective vulnerability.[3] Most favor the idea of Holbourn,[4] that contusion results from friction between the brain and the rough surfaced floors of the anterior and middle fossae of the skull.[5]

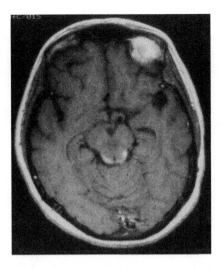

Figure 6.1 Deafness resulted from these bilateral contusions of the inferior colliculi.

The brain can also be sloshed against folds of dura. The edge of the falx cerebri sits above the corpus callosum. If blunt head trauma bounces the brain against the relatively fixed and often ossified falx, the corpus callosum can be damaged. Occasionally, very interesting contusion syndromes occur. The brainstem can be whipped back against the tentorium, whose firm dural edge can contuse the inferior colliculi (Figure 6.1). Symmetric damage to these structures can result in total deafness as the only permanent sequela of the accident.[6] In these cases, selective vulnerability is simply a matter of a particular part of the brain being located near a portion of dura, against which it can be flung.

VASCULAR DISEASE

Selective vulnerability in vascular disease is related to structural features and simple physics. In varied settings, authors have applied the *border zone concept* to explain selective vulnerability to cerebral infarction.

The anterior and middle cerebral arteries supply different territories. There is a region between their areas of primary supply where flow to the end vessels is tenuous. Hence, we commonly see severe hypotension resulting in infarction in the border zone. In some cases, the affected border zone is in the cortex (between cortical branches); in some, in the white matter (between deep penetrating branches); and in some, it is in both. This phenomenon is usually compared to a sprinkler system in which the pressure is too low to water the area where the supply of two spouts usually overlap. (The term "watershed," often applied to arterial border zone infarction, is an inappropriate usage. A watershed is an area on the border of two drainage systems of streams and rivers. For example, there is a watershed in Ohio; in one direction, the water drains to Lake Erie and, in the other direction, to the Mississippi River system. The proper analogy in neurology would be an area on one side of which blood drains toward one major vein and on the other side of which it drains toward another vein or venous sinus.)

Infarctions in the border zone are not always due to global hypotension. Patients with malignant hypertension are sometimes treated so vigorously that the blood pressure can drop in hours or less from 250/120 to 140/70, for example. This sudden decrement in blood pressure is, in effect, relative hypotension, and it can cause border zone infarction. If a carotid artery is occluded, collateral circulation may adequately supply the ipsilateral hemisphere except in the border zone. Major border zone territories can be affected by embolism from the heart. Microemboliflow through the cerebral circulation before occluding the small distal vessels.[7] Hence, the resulting tiny brain infarcts tend to occur in arterial border zone areas.

The border zones are important in premature infants. *Periventricular leukomalacia* is a term applied to necrotic areas in the cerebral white matter near the lateral ventricles. The lesions are presumed to be a form of hypoxic-ischemic injury at the deep border zones of the major cortical arteries. Incomplete development of the distal branches, penetrating from the surface arteries, is apparently responsible for the territorial vulnerability.[8–10]

The preferential locations for cervical artery dissections are explained by structural and mechanical factors.[11] Deceleration injury causes dissection of the vertebral artery after the vessel emerges from the protection of the transverse foramen of C2. Vulnerability is particular to this mobile area of the vertebral artery. The vessel is otherwise protected both where it is immobilized by the dura intracranially and where it is immobile as it passes through the cervical vertebrae in its ascent. Where a vessel can be whipped, its wall can be torn. Likewise the deceleration of the carotid artery causes dissection where the vessel is mobile, high in the neck before it enters the carotid canal. Internal carotid artery dissection, which occurs in the absence of overt trauma, has been attributed to head twisting and compression of the artery against a long styloid process.[12,13]

There are geometrically preferred areas for the development of atherosclerosis of the brain-supplying arteries.[14] Vascular branching points such as those of the cervical carotid arteries are predisposed. The meeting of the vertebral arteries at the basilar artery is also a selectively vulnerable juncture. It is the outer walls of the vessels which show more atherosclerosis. These are the areas where there is relatively weak flow, weak shear strain, and weak frictional force on the endothelium. The areas with less atherosclerosis are those with unidirectional axial flow and high shear stress. Observations on humans and experiments on animals have supported these general statements. For example, surgically created high-flow fistulas develop little atherosclerosis.

Berry aneurysms are an interesting subject in selective vulnerability. Why are the intracranial vessels affected almost exclusively, and why are certain sites in the brain's arterial supply disproportionately affected?

Saccular aneurysms only rarely occur extracranially. The propensity of the brain's arteries to this disease can be explained by the structure of the cerebral vessels. The media and the adventitia are thin compared to other arteries. Furthermore, the elastica of intracranial arteries is diminished compared to that present in other arterial systems.[15,16] Specifically, the external elastic lamina is virtually absent and the internal elastic lamina is sparse. Overall, the vessel walls are translucent and weak compared to the more elastic and durable peripheral arteries. Thus it is understandable that the weak, thin-walled subarachnoid vessels have the propensity to develop saccular aneurysms.

Not all sites in the cerebral arteries are equally vulnerable to the development of berry aneurysms. They occur primarily where arteries fork. These aneurysms are found typically at the bifurcation of the middle cerebral artery, the bifurcation of the internal carotid, the juncture of the internal carotid with the posterior communicating artery, the connection of the anterior communicating artery and the anterior cerebral artery, and the bifurcation of the basilar artery. Why do aneurysms occur at arterial branching points? In neonates, one often finds disruption of the internal elastic lamina at branching points.[15] In other words, the already flimsy cerebral arteries are even weaker at the junctures and thus more vulnerable to hemodynamic stress. Although wall weakness at branching sites is present in babies, infants rarely have berry aneurysms. Stehbens goes so far as to say that, under age 13, the "incidence is virtually nil."[16] Aneurysm, in other words, is an acquired lesion. Congenitally weak sites in the walls of arteries, with decades of hemodynamic stress, slowly develop the out-pouching that we call aneurysm.

INFECTIOUS DISEASE

In endocarditis, the mechanism of formation of aneurysms and the selective vulnerability of vessels to them differs.[17] Emboli from the inflamed heart valves tend to lodge in more distal vessels because the emboli are ordinarily not large enough to occlude a carotid or middle cerebral artery. Thus, a mycotic aneurysm forms when the inflammatory process spreads from the embolic fragment to the adjacent wall of the plugged distal artery. Hence unlike the typically proximal berry aneurysm, the characteristic mycotic aneurysm occurs distally (Figure 6.2A).

The locations of hematogenous brain abscesses are also understood by their embolic origins. Tiny infectious fragments or bacteria are thought to lodge in the subcortical end arteries at the gray–white junction, where they become the seeds of abscesses (Figure 6.2B).[18,19] Other areas of brain are thought to have less of an end arteriole pattern. In other words, brain regions where there is more microvascular collateral flow are relatively spared. The most common

(A)

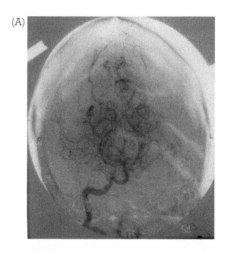

(B)

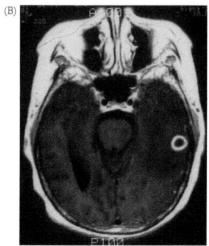

Figure 6.2 Selective vulnerability in infectious disease. (A) A mycotic cerebral aneurysm. Unlike berry aneurysm, it is typically distal. (B) When septicemia seeds the brain, the abscess characteristically occurs in the subcortical area.

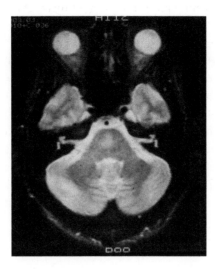

Figure 6.3 Selective vulnerability in infectious disease. *Listeria* rhombencephalitis. The brainstem is vulnerable to this infection.

location of these microabscesses is the area supplied by the distal middle cerebral artery branches.

Herpes simplex encephalitis disproportionately affects the medial temporal lobe and nearby structures. This selective vulnerability has intrigued doctors, who have offered ideas to explain it.[20] One theory was that the virus enters the nose and spreads through the olfactory pathway to its cerebral connections, which are close to the medial temporal lobe and the frontal lobe. A later concept was that a virus, latent in the trigeminal ganglion, spreads through branches of the trigeminal nerve to the dura of the anterior and middle cranial fossae and somehow spreads to the adjacent brain. A third hypothesis is that the tissue of the limbic system has a particular vulnerability to this virus and that the method of spread to the brain is not a primary determinant of localization. All of these ideas are speculative.

There are many other examples of selective vulnerability in infectious disease (see Figure 6.3).

TUMOR

Hematogenous metastases preferentially occur in a distribution similar to that of embolic microabscesses. The same mechanism that explains the preferred location of brain abscesses is invoked to explain the disproportionate number of brain metastases which occur in the subcortical white matter (cortical gray–white junction). Posner states that the selective vulnerability of the gray–white junction results from it being the site where arterioles, penetrating from cortical surface vessels, first separate into capillary beds.[21,22]

SPONDYLOSIS

The cervical and lumbar spines are vulnerable to spondylotic radiculopathy and myelopathy because they are much more mobile than the thoracic spine. The spinal movement, over decades, leads to wear and tear of discs, bones, and ligaments. The thoracic spine has less spondylosis because the rib cage limits its mobility. The importance of the rib cage is indicated by the distribution of herniated thoracic discs. When thoracic disc herniations do occur, they are usually found below T8, where the ribs provide less structural support.[23] Thoracic disc herniation is so much less common than that at the cervical and lumbar levels that it was not well described until mid-century.

HYPOXIA

Vulnerability to hypoxia/anoxia varies between gross brain regions, cell types, and even microscopic territories. Neurons are more vulnerable than glial cells. Cerebral cortex is more vulnerable than the thalamus, which is more vulnerable than the brainstem. Within the cortex, layers 3–5 are most vulnerable. Of all the regions of cerebral cortex, the Sommer sector of the hippocampus is extremely sensitive to anoxia. It is difficult to separate whether nonvascular or vascular vulnerability determines the areas likely to be affected in global hypoxic/ischemic encephalopathies. Does the preferential damage to cerebral cortical layers 3–5 derive from the one or the other mechanism? The relative resistance of the brainstem is hard to explain on the basis of vascular supply. Totally unexplained is the preferential involvement of cerebral white matter in delayed anoxic leukoencephalopathy.

TOXIC/METABOLIC DISEASES

Characteristic brain areas are affected in a given metabolic insult. The apparent specificity of such lesions often leads to the discovery and naming of a disease. Only later comes recognition that the vulnerable locations vary from the brain of one individual to another.

Central pontine myelinolysis is a good example of the complexity of selective vulnerability. There was much discussion about the center of the pons, about what made it selectively vulnerable. Eventually, extrapontine myelinolysis was recognized.[24] The discussion then turned to all of the involved territories. What commonality made them vulnerable? There has been no satisfactory explanation to date. All that can be said is that there are multiple territories vulnerable to this

disease and that the distribution of the disease depends on the relative vulner-
abilities of these territories in a given individual. As noted above, there was much
speculation about the special vulnerability of the center of the basis pontis. Little
noticed were the rare case reports of myelinolysis occurring symmetrically in the
lateral pons and sparing the center of the pons. Information from our laboratory
suggests that the anatomy of the center of the pons should not be expected to provide a simple answer to the question of selective vulnerability. Figure 6.4 shows

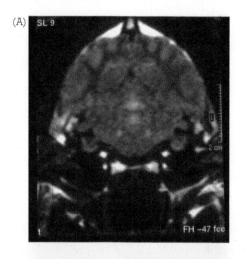

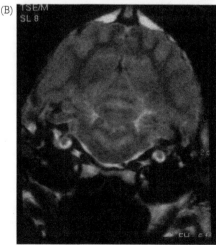

Figure 6.4 Magnetic resonance imaging (MRI) scans from an experimental
animal. (A) Pontine myelinolysis begins symmetrically off center in this particular
individual. (B) On a subsequent scan, the lesions have "fused" into a single central
pontine lesion.

evoling canine myelinolysis. Initially, the image shows symmetric paracentral lesions. Only on a subsequent day does the image show the lesions "fused" into a pontine lesion centered on the midline. Perhaps the center is not a simple clue to central pontine disease.

We do not know the reason for selective vulnerability in metabolic diseases. How can we explain methanol affecting the putamen and relatively sparing the globus pallidus (Figure 6.5A)? Who can explain nutritional cerebellar degeneration affecting the midline anterior-superior vermis while sparing the inferior vermis and the hemispheres (Figure 6.6A)? Why is the

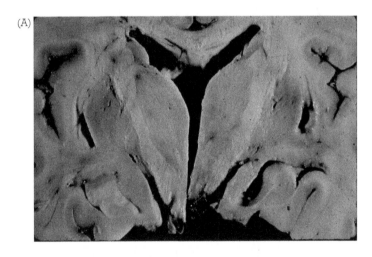

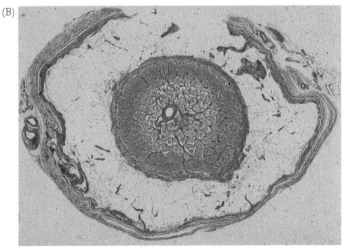

Figure 6.5 Selective vulnerability occurs in methanol poisoning. (A) illustrates the vulnerability of the putamina, which are cavitated. (B) shows the selective vulnerability of the anterior visual system with demyelination in the center of the optic nerve.

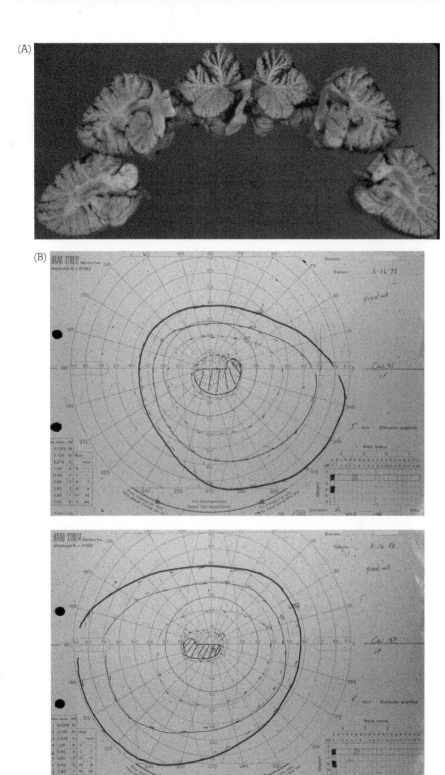

Figure 6.6 Selective vulnerability in nutritional disease. (A) Atrophy limited to the anterior superior vermis. (B) Cecocentral scotomas of nutritional optic neuropathy are similar in the two eyes.

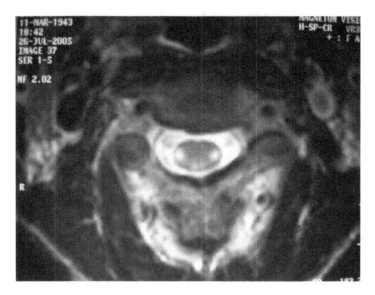

Figure 6.7 Selective vulnerability in subacute combined degeneration of the spinal cord with characteristic posterior and lateral column lesions.

papillomacular bundle vulnerable in nutritional optic nerve disease compared to the axons of other retinal ganglion cells (Figure 6.6B)? Why are the posterior and lateral columns of the spinal cord selectively vulnerable in subacute combined degeneration (Figure 6.7)? There can be no doubt of the selective vulnerability in these diseases, but, in general, the basis of the vulnerability is a mystery.

DEMYELINATIVE DISEASE

Microscopically, multiple sclerosis is a perivenular inflammatory demyelinative disease. Grossly, there is a disproportionate number of plaques in the periventricular white matter. Residents always wonder about this selective vulnerability. Why do these lesions (Dawson's fingers) occur near the cerebral ventricles? The answer is simply that this perivenular disease occurs where there are veins and that many veins pass through the periventricular white matter en route to the larger subependymal veins (Figure 6.8).

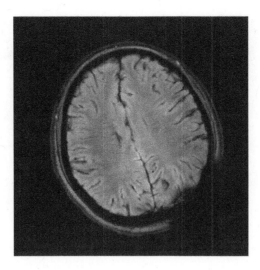

Figure 6.8 This magnetic resonance image (MRI) shows linear veins heading toward the lateral ventricles. It demonstrates why a perivenous disease (multiple sclerosis) tends to cause lesions perpendicular to the ventricles.

NEUROMUSCULAR DISEASE

In neuralgic amyotrophy, some nerves derived from the brachial plexus are more likely to be affected. Vulnerable are the long thoracic nerve and the anterior interosseous nerve. The radial nerve is typically spared. Unknown is the reason for the preferential involvement.

In myasthenia gravis, there is incompletely understood vulnerability of the levator palpebrae, extraocular muscles, and other bulbar-innervated muscles. In the limbs, there are interesting patterns of selective vulnerability as well. Robert Leshner has observed that the neck extensors, foot dorsiflexors, triceps, wrist flexors, and finger extensors are disproportionately affected (Robert Leshner, MD, in conversation, 2016). Campbell and colleagues have documented the selective vulnerability of the triceps.[25]

Undoubtedly genetic in origin is the remarkably selective vulnerability in muscular dystrophies. In facioscapulohumeral dystrophy, for example, a certain muscle may be severely affected on the right and left while a neighboring muscle is little affected.

There are many puzzles in diseases of muscle. Inclusion body myositis is a good example. The very selective weakness of finger and wrist flexors and the quadriceps is characteristic and unexplained. In thyroid ophthalmopathy, there is no understanding of the selective vulnerability of the inferior rectus

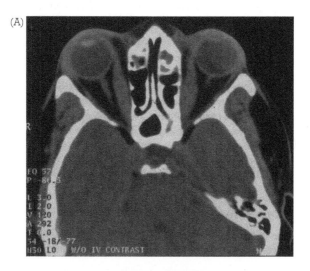

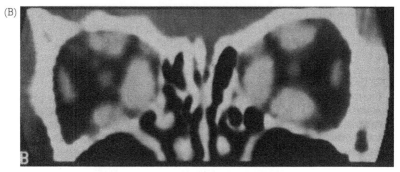

Figure 6.9 Selective vulnerability in Graves's ophthalmopathy. The medial rectus is disproportionately affected compared to the lateral rectus.

and medial rectus (Figure 6.9). The pattern of weakness in toxic muscle disease is puzzling in its interindividual proximal or distal predominant pattern. Most often the primary vulnerability is in the proximal muscles. I have seen, however, a case of simvastatin myopathy with selective involvement of distal muscles. In metabolic myopathy, like vitamin E deficiency, there are scattered necrotic muscle fibers. We have no idea why one muscle fiber is severely affected and another is not.

CONCLUSION

Disease of the CNS can selectively affect brain systems, brain structures, or brain regions. Selective system involvement is clear in degenerative diseases such as amyotrophic lateral sclerosis. Selective structure vulnerability occurs in carbon monoxide's effect on the globus pallidus (Figure 6.10). Selective region involvement is found in myelinolysis. In the pons myelinolysis can affect multiple neural systems and structures. In other words, myelinolysis affects a territory rather than a neural structure or system.

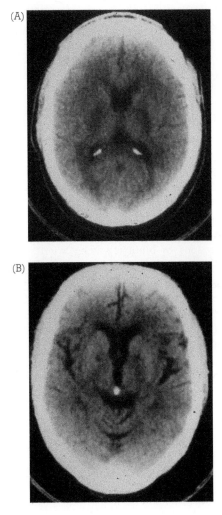

Figure 6.10 Carbon monoxide poisoning. (A) Symmetric globus pallidus lesions in a patient found unresponsive in his rooming house. A few days after I saw him, I learned that his roommate had also been admitted to the hospital. I found the roommate awake on a medical ward. He had smaller globus pallidus lesions, shown in (B).

REFERENCES

1. Klatzo I. Cécile and Oskar Vogt: the visionaries of modern neuroscience. *Acta Neurochir Suppl.* 2002;80:VI–XIII, 1–130.

2. Denny-Brown D, Russell WR. Experimental cerebral concussion. *Brain.* 1941;64(pts. 2–3):93–163.

3. Huang HM, Lee MC, Lee SY, Chiu WT, Pan LC, Chen CT. Finite element analysis of brain contusion: an indirect impact study. *Med Biol Eng Comput.* 2000;38(3):253–259.

4. Holbourn AHS. Mechanics of head injuries. *Lancet.* 1943;242(6267):438–441.

5. Ommaya AK, Grubb RL, Naumann RA. Coup and contre-coup injury: observations on the mechanics of visible brain injuries in the rhesus monkey. *J Neurosurg.* 1971;35(5):503–516.

6. Jani NN, Laureno R, Mark AS, Brewer CC. Deafness after bilateral midbrain contusion: a correlation of magnetic resonance imaging with auditory brain stem evoked responses. *Neurosurgery.* 1991;29(1):106–8-9.

7. Bergui M, Castagno D, D'Agata F, Cicerale A, Anselmino M, Maria Ferrio F, Giustetto C, et al. Selective vulnerability of cortical border zone to microembolic infarct. *Stroke.* 2015;46(7):1864–1869.

8. Banker BQ, Larroche JC. Periventricular leukomalacia of infancy. A form of neonatal anoxic encephalopathy. *Arch Neurol.* 1962;7:386–410.

9. Khwaja O, Volpe JJ. Pathogenesis of cerebral white matter injury of prematurity. *Arch Dis Child - Fetal Neonatal Ed.* 2007;93(2):F153–F161.

10. De Reuck J. The human periventricular arterial blood supply and the anatomy of cerebral infarctions. *Eur Neurol.* 1971;5(6):321–334.

11. Caplan LR. Dissections of brain-supplying arteries. *Nat Clin Pract Neurol.* 2008;4(1):34–42.

12. Raser JM, Mullen MT, Kasner SE, Cucchiara BL, Messé SR. Cervical carotid artery dissection is associated with styloid process length. *Neurology.* 2011;77(23):2061–2066.

13. Muthusami P, Kesavadas C, Sylaja PN, Thomas B, Harsha KJ, Kapilamoorthy TR. Implicating the long styloid process in cervical carotid artery dissection. *Neuroradiology.* 2013;55(7):861–867.

14. Malek AM, Alper SL, Izumo S. Hemodynamic shear stress and its role in atherosclerosis. *JAMA.* 1999;282(21):2035–2042.

15. Stehbens WE. Pathology and pathogenesis of intracranial berry aneurysms. *Neurol Res.* 1990;12(1):29–34.

16. Stehbens WE. *Pathology of the cerebral blood vessels.* St. Louis, MO: Mosby; 1972.

17. Roach MR, Drake CG. Ruptured cerebral aneurysms caused by micro-organisms. *N Engl J Med.* 1965;273(5):240–244.

18. Adams RD, Sidman RL. *Introduction to neuropathology.* New York: McGraw Hill; 1968.

19. Adams RD, Victor M. *Principles of neurology.* New York: McGraw Hill; 1977.

20. Damasio AR, Van Hoesen GW. The limbic system and the localisation of herpes simplex encephalitis. *J Neurol Neurosurg Psychiatry.* 1985;48(4):297–301.

21. Delattre JY, Krol G, Thaler HT, Posner JB. Distribution of brain metastases. *Arch Neurol.* 1988;45(7):741–744.

22. Posner JB. *Neurologic complications of cancer.* Philadelphia, PA: F.A. Davis; 1995.
23. Rao RD, Smuck M, eds. *Orthopedic knowledge update: spine 4.* Rosemont, IL: American Academy of Orthopedic Surgeons; 2012.
24. Wright DG, Laureno R, Victor M. Pontine and extrapontine myelinolysis. *Brain.* 1979;102(2):361–385.
25. Domingo CA, Landau ME, Campbell WW. Selective triceps muscle weakness in myasthenia gravis is underrecognized. *J Clin Neuromuscul Dis.* 2016;18(2):103–104.

7

Normalization

R apid normalization of a systemic medical disorder can cause neurologic disturbance and disease. Treatment of diabetes, uremia, and certain electrolyte disorders are examples. Stopping regular use of a medication would seem to bring the body to a more normal (unmedicated) state, but, in some cases, there are neurologic complications to rapid discontinuation. Likewise, a withdrawal syndrome can follow sudden cessation of a regularly used nonmedicinal chemical. Although alcohol is the best known example, sudden abstinence from other habitually used chemicals can cause neurologic withdrawal phenomena. Not all normalization disorders are chemical or metabolic. Rapid correction of increased intracranial pressure or rapid lowering of severe arterial hypertension are examples.

RENAL FAILURE AND ELECTROLYTE DISORDERS

The rapid correction of uremia by dialysis can cause neurologic deterioration.[1] This dialysis disequilibrium syndrome typically occurs toward the end of or after a dialysis treatment. The neurologic deterioration can be manifest as headache, delirium, confusion, obtundation, and/or seizures. When urea rapidly declines in the blood, the high concentration of urea in the brain draws in water and the brain swells. Computed tomography (CT) scans have confirmed the association of the disequilibrium syndrome with brain swelling. The increased brain water content with rapid dialysis has been demonstrated in animal experiments. The "reverse urea effect" with cerebral edema may not be the total explanation for the disequilibrium symptoms, but it is the best-defined aspect of the syndrome. This disorder can be avoided by moderating the pace of dialysis. Widespread recognition of the risk of rapid normalization has made dialysis-induced encephalopathy uncommon today. Earlier initiation of dialysis has also lessened this adverse effect. In the early years of dialysis, the treatment was not started until the patient was grossly uremic. Now, when dialysis is initiated before uremia is so advanced, the potential for a massive, rapid drop in blood parameters has diminished.

Rapid normalization or improvement of electrolyte derangements can produce neurologic disorders.[2] Most dramatic are the sodium problems, hyponatremia and hypernatremia. Under special circumstances, correction of hypokalemia can also precipitate neurologic worsening.

The encephalopathy of hypernatremia is minimized by osmoprotective mechanisms. Brain cells take in K^+ and accumulate amines and polyols, all of which increase intracellular osmolality. It takes days for these intracellular osmolytes to accumulate and thereby balance the osmolality of the brain cells with the osmolality of the hypernatremic extracellular milieu. When hypernatremia is corrected, the intracellular osmolytes cannot dissipate quickly. If the serum sodium is rapidly lowered, water is drawn into the brain, and cerebral edema results. Such iatrogenic brain swelling can be avoided by lowering serum sodium no more than 0.5 mEq/L per hour.[2]

In hyponatremia, rapid correction can cause a distinctive brain disease, myelinolysis (Figurer 7.1).[3] This term was selected to denote the relative sparing of neurons and axons and the preferential damage to myelin in the brain lesions. Because the disease was originally discovered in the center of the pons, it was designated central pontine myelinolysis. Before long, symmetric extrapontine lesions were observed to be associated with the pontine disease in some cases. Eventually CT and magnetic resonance imaging (MRI) scans revealed that striatal or thalamic lesions could occur in the absence of a pontine lesion. Due to the variation in territories affected, some are inclined to use a term that emphasizes pathogenesis over anatomic areas affected. "Osmotic myelinolysis" is one such term. To minimize the chances of myelinolysis occurring following correction of hyponatremia, the serum sodium rise should be limited to 6 mEq/L per 24 hours whenever possible.

Correction of hypokalemia can also cause a neurologic problem. Hypokalemia protects a hypocalcemic patient from tetany. Thus, when hypocalcemia coexists with hypokalemia, correction of hypokalemia can precipitate tetany.

DIABETES

Insulin therapy for diabetes mellitus was first used in 1922. The treatment was noted to be followed by the subacute onset of polyneuropathy in some

(A)

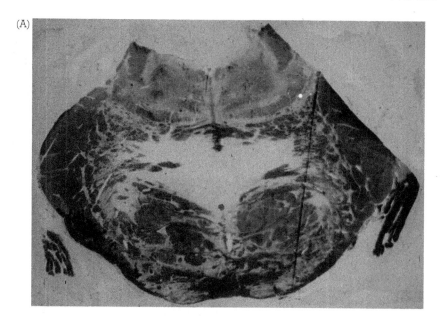

(B)

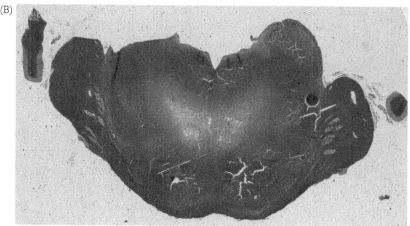

Figure 7.1 Central pontine myelinolysis following rapid correction of hyponatremia in the human (A) and dog (B).

patients.[4] Originally called "insulin neuritis," this complication has been more recently termed "treatment-induced neuropathy of diabetes."[5] Somehow, the relatively rapid normalization of blood sugar results in damage to small unmyelinated sensory and autonomic peripheral nerve fibers. The greater the drop in one's glycosylated hemoglobin (HbA1C) over the early months of treatment, the greater the risk of developing the painful polyneuropathy. At an extreme, a 3-month fall of more than 4% in HbA1C is associated with an 80% risk of treatment-induced neuropathy.[5] Exactly how normalization of blood sugar causes neuropathy is unknown. The prognosis for eventual improvement is good. Treatment-induced neuropathy in diabetes has been underrecognized because many cases have been assumed to be a form of the common, distal, sensorimotor diabetic polyneuropathy.

There was a time when an extremely low pH in diabetic ketoacidosis was considered so life-threatening that bicarbonate was given to promptly improve the acidosis. Infusion of bicarbonate would raise the pH by buffering protons. In the process of improving systemic acidosis, the treatment would generate water (H_2O) and carbon dioxide (CO_2). Since CO_2 readily diffuses into the spinal fluid, the well-intended therapy would often result in cerebrospinal fluid (CSF) acidosis: this treatment could change a profoundly acidotic awake patient into an obtunded person with improved blood pH. By relying on insulin and avoiding bicarbonate in the therapy of diabetic ketoacidosis, doctors have eliminated this iatrogenic form of stupor and coma.[6]

In severe diabetic ketoacidosis, rapid lowering of blood sugar can result in cerebral edema.[7] Death related to diabetic ketoacidosis associated cerebral edema was first reported in 1936.[8] Later, increased spinal fluid pressure was documented during the treatment of this disorder.[8] At one point a "wave of cerebral edema . . . occurred mainly in young patients receiving large amounts of hypotonic fluids given by exuberant house staff in major medical centers."[9] During correction of hyperglycemia, one avoids this cerebral edema by not using hypotonic intravenous fluid and not lowering plasma osmolality too rapidly.

In nonketotic hyperglycemia, similar caution in correction can protect patients from iatrogenic cerebral edema. Initial documentation of treatment-related brain swelling came in dog experiments. Rapid lowering of high blood sugar led to a rise in CSF pressure. Furthermore, CSF measurements of fructose and sorbitol led to the idea that an increase of intracellular polyols during hyperglycemia predisposed to cerebral edema during treatment. It was soon thereafter shown that cerebral edema could complicate treatment of nonketotic hyperglycemia in the human.[8,10]

Children are especially vulnerable to cerebral edema in the treatment of hyperglycemia. In addition the child's brain cannot tolerate the modest swelling that an adult can because the young brain, yet to atrophy, has little intracranial space to accommodate expansion.

REFEEDING SYNDROME

After prolonged starvation, resumption of eating can cause a multisystem disease.[11] The neuromuscular manifestations are a combination of polyneuropathy and myopathy due to electrolyte derangements such as hypophosphatemia and hypokalemia. The normalization of nutritional intake produces the electrolyte changes that precipitate the neurologic problems. The refeeding syndrome is primarily a problem of liberated prisoners of war.[11]

INTRACRANIAL PRESSURE

Rapid decompression of the CNS can cause deleterious effects. In cases of brain tumor with papilledema, optic neuropathy can result from surgical relief of elevated intracranial pressure.[12] With shunting for hydrocephalus, a precipitous drop in ventricular pressure can also lead to permanent vision loss. These patients with long-standing papilledema develop optic nerve damage from a poorly understood ischemic process. A capillary network supplies the optic nerve head, which is continuously subject to both intra-ocular and intracranial pressures. A sudden drop in intracranial pressure is more likely to affect the optic nerve head adversely in the presence of low arterial blood pressure or high intraocular pressure.[13] Neither of these variables, however, need be present for a CSF pressure drop to cause optic nerve ischemia.

Tumor and hydrocephalus are not the only settings in which loss of vision can result from precipitous lowering of CSF pressure by shunting. The same complication can occur with sudden normalization of pressure in idiopathic intracranial hypertension or other "pseudotumor cerebri" cases. These nonhy-drocephalic cases ordinarily do not receive shunts unless there is already visual loss. Thus one might postulate that any postoperative loss of vision could be due to progression of the original process. However, the sudden deterioration of vision resembles the precipitous decline in vision after shunting of hydrocephalus. Iatrogenic visual loss can occur from the sudden normalization of high CSF pressure of any cause.

ARTERIAL HYPERTENSION

Rapid lowering of high blood pressure can damage the brain (Figure 7.2). When treating severe hypertension, one may lower the blood pressure more than intended, and the relative hypotension may cause bilateral ischemic brain damage. To avoid this complication, one should lower blood pressure no more than 20% over a 24-hour period. Additionally, when there is acute cerebral infarction, sudden marked lowering of blood pressure can make the stroke worse. Thus, one tolerates hypertension in the setting of fresh stroke.[14,15]

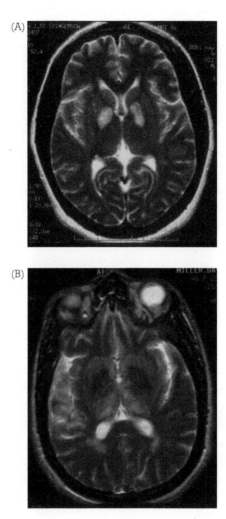

Figure 7.2 Overly aggressive correction of severe hypertension can result in ischemic brain injury. In one patient, the basal ganglia were disproportionately damaged (A). In another patient, the thalami were disproportionately affected (B).

NORMALIZATION BY WITHDRAWAL
OF CHEMICALS AND DRUGS

It was not always known that an intoxicated person could suffer ill effects from ceasing alcohol consumption. Getting back to the normal alcohol-free state, it seemed, would be good. As astute an observer as Mark Twain portrayed the hallucinations of Huckleberry Finn's father as a manifestation of inebriation.

In medical circles, the role of abstinence was much debated well into the 20th century. It was the work of Maurice Victor and Raymond Adams that made the alcohol withdrawal syndromes obvious to all.[16]

The alcohol abstinence syndromes imprinted the idea of withdrawal disorders on the medical community. Analogous withdrawal syndromes occur with other sedating medications.[17,18] After chronic use of paraldehyde, barbiturates, or benzodiazepines, withdrawal seizures and other manifestations can follow precipitous stoppage. The latency to withdrawal symptoms varies with the half-life of the medication. Because alprazolam's half-life can be less than 12 hours, withdrawal seizures can occur soon after the last dose. On the other hand, diazepam has such a long half-life that withdrawal seizures can occur more than a week after the medication has been stopped. The sleeping medication zolpidem is in a different pharmacologic family, but when it has been taken regularly in excessive doses, its precipitous withdrawal can cause restlessness and seizures.

Other chemicals chronically taken for pleasure can cause abstinence problems. Heroin, cocaine, synthetic cathinones, and synthetic cannabinoids each have their own abstinence syndromes. There are many other examples. Furthermore, the ever-changing menu of habituating and addicting chemicals means that new withdrawal syndromes will emerge.

Withdrawal of medications other than hypnotics and sedatives can result in neurologic disorders. Abrupt cessation of the antispasticity medicine baclofen (oral or intrathecal) can result in confusion, agitation, seizures, perceptual problems, and other psychiatric symptoms. Stopping doxepin, a tricyclic antidepressant, can cause delirium. Dyskinesia can be a neuroleptic discontinuation reaction. Precipitous cessation of gabapentin use can cause anxiety and other symptoms. Suddenly discontinuing propranolol can cause headaches.

Some withdrawal phenomena are due in part to a flare of the disease which a medication had been suppressing. Acetazolamide and furosemide have been used to treat hydrocephalus in infants. Abrupt stoppage of the medications could be followed by sudden head enlargement (Arnold Gale, MD, in conversation, c. 1988). Suddenly stopping dexamethasone being used for treatment of the brain edema of multiple brain metastases can lead to florid cerebral edema. A similar response can follow the withdrawal of steroid medication being used for tuberculous meningitis. In the absence of neurologic disease abrupt stoppage of high doses of corticosteroid medicine also can cause intracranial hypertension.

The foregoing are only a few examples of neurologic syndromes due to normalization by withdrawal of medication. In general, the higher the dose and the longer the use, the more likely discontinuation will result in symptoms. As new medications are developed, new withdrawal syndromes will be discovered. Avoiding a sudden return to the normal, unmedicated state will lessen the chances of withdrawal symptoms.

STROKE

Medication withdrawal can lead to stroke. For example, rebound hypercoagulability after discontinuation of warfarin can lead to ischemic stroke.[19] Withdrawal of aspirin can similarly be followed by a stroke.[20] Withdrawal of clopidogrel can do the same. I cared for a middle-aged woman who had been chronically taking vitamin E daily. She was instructed to stop taking it days prior to cosmetic facial surgery. Before the surgery could be done, there ensued, without other explanation, lenticulostriate artery occlusion with severe hemiplegia. These prothrombotic withdrawal effects are not limited to patients with preexisting hypercoagulable states.

Stroke can result from rapid normalization of deviant hematologic parameters to which the body has become accustomed. I remember a patient who was doing well with a stable platelet count of 20,000. In preparation for oral surgery, dexamethasone was prescribed to treat the thrombocytopenia. The platelet count did rapidly rise toward normal. Before oral surgery could be performed, the patient had a cerebral infarction. There was no explanation for this stroke other than the rapid rise in the platelet count to 130,000. Severe chronic anemia is another situation in which rapid normalization can be damaging. I saw a young woman with sickle cell anemia in whom transfusion doubled the hematocrit to a normal level in a matter of hours. The intent was to improve the hematocrit preoperatively. Promptly, the patient developed cerebral infarction. There was no other explanation for the stroke. Although regular modest transfusion can prevent strokes in sickle cell anemia patients, aggressive transfusion can suddenly result in a dangerous rise in blood viscosity.

EPILEPSY

"Forced normalization" is a term that was proposed more than half a century ago. It refers to a concept that psychosis can result from rather sudden control of seizures in patients who have had long-standing uncontrolled epilepsy. I do not recall seeing a patient in whom achievement of seizure control caused psychosis. Nevertheless, hallucinations, paranoia and other manifestations have been observed.[21]

FINAL COMMENTS

1. At certain hospitals, at certain times, resident physician jargon has indicated a macho attitude about aggressive treatments. "Hot salt" has referred to 3% saline infusion for rapidly correcting hyponatremia. "Slam him" with one medicine or another has referred to rapidly giving a lot. It is best to avoid this glib language.

2. The more severe and the more prolonged an abnormality, the more likely its correction can cause neurologic manifestations. Such normalization phenomena occur in disorders of blood chemistry, arterial blood pressure, intracranial pressure, and the cellular elements of blood. Many of these problems are iatrogenic. Often the doctor better serves the patient by tempering his urge to treat quickly.

REFERENCES

1. Silver SM, DeSimone JA, Smith DA, Sterns RH. Dialysis disequilibrium syndrome (DDS) in the rat: role of the "reverse urea effect." *Kidney Int.* 1992;42(1):161–166.

2. Laureno R. Neurologic syndromes accompanying electrolyte disorders. In: Goetz CG, Tanner CM, Aminoff MJ, eds., *Systemic diseases, vol. 1.* Amsterdam: Elsevier Science Publishers; 1993:545–573. *Handbook of Clinical Neurology,* vol. 63.

3. Laureno R. Central pontine myelinolysis following rapid correction of hyponatremia. *Ann Neurol.* 1983;13(3):232–242.

4 Ellenberg M. Diabetic neuropathy precipitating after institution of diabetic control. *Am J Med Sci.* 1958;236(4):466–471.

5. Gibbons CH, Freeman R. Treatment-induced diabetic neuropathy: a reversible painful autonomic neuropathy. *Ann Neurol.* 2010;67(4):534–541.

6. Posner JB, Plum F. Spinal-fluid pH and neurologic symptoms in systemic acidosis. *N Engl J Med.* 1967;277(12):605–613.

7. Silver SM, Clark EC, Schroeder BM, Sterns RH. Pathogenesis of cerebral edema after treatment of diabetic ketoacidosis. *Kidney Int.* 1997;51(4):1237–1244.

8. Duck SC, Weldon VV, Pagliara AS, Haymond MW. Cerebral edema complicating therapy for diabetic ketoacidosis. *Diabetes.* 1976;25(2):111–115.

9. Cahill GF. Diabetic coma: ketoacidotic and hyperosmolar. *New England J Med.* 1982;307:568.

10. Maccario M, Messis CP. Cerebral oedema complicating treated non-ketotic hyperglycaemia. *Lancet (London, England).* 1969;2(7616):352–353.

11. Hearing SD. Refeeding syndrome. *BMJ.* 2004;328(7445):908–909.

12. Beck RW, Greenberg HS. Post-decompression optic neuropathy. *J Neurosurg.* 1985;63(2):196–199.

13. Corbett JJ. Neuro-ophthalmologic complications of hydrocephalus and shunting procedures. *Semin Neurol.* 1986;6(2):111–123.

14. Castillo J, Leira R, García MM, Serena J, Blanco M, Dávalos A. Blood pressure decrease during the acute phase of ischemic stroke is associated with brain injury and poor stroke outcome. *Stroke*. 2004;35(2):520–526.

15. Graham DI. Ischaemic brain damage of cerebral perfusion failure type after treatment of severe hypertension. *Br Med J*. 1975;4(5999):739.

16. Victor M, Adams RD. The effect of alcohol on the nervous system. *Res Publ Assoc Res Nerv Ment Dis*. 1953;32:526–573.

17. Isbell H, Altschul S, Kornetsky CH, Eisenman AJ, Flanary HG, Fraser HF. Chronic barbiturate intoxication; an experimental study. *Arch Neurol Psychiatry*. 1950;64(1):1–28.

18. Kalinowsky LB. Convulsions in nonepileptic patients on withdrawal of barbiturates, alcohol and other drugs. *Arch NeurPsych*. 1942;48(6):946–956.

19. Schanbacher CF, Bennett RG. Postoperative stroke after stopping warfarin for cutaneous surgery. *Dermatol Surg*. 2000;26(8):785–789.

20. Doutremepuich C, Aguejouf O, Desplat V, Eizayaga FX. Aspirin discontinuation syndromes: clinical implications of basic research studies. *Am J Cardiovasc Drugs*. 2013;13(6):377–384.

21. Pakalnis A, Drake ME, John K, Kellum JB. Forced normalization. Acute psychosis after seizure control in seven patients. *Arch Neurol*. 1987;44(3):289–292.

8

Asymptomatic Disease

A symptomatic disease can be discovered by routine physical examination or by diagnostic tests that have been ordered for some unrelated reason. Discovery of asymptomatic disease is not always accidental. We sometimes search for asymptomatic brain disease. Such testing can be prompted by the family history, the patient's personal history, or the clinical situation. After an asymptomatic condition has been found, one must decide how to use the information. Judgment, in such cases, can be difficult.

DISCOVERY BY ROUTINE EXAMINATION

An internist or a pediatrician may notice asymptomatic disease from cutaneous clues like café au lait spots or adenoma sebaceum. These doctors may notice the myopathic facies of an asymptomatic dystrophy or the distal wasting of a hereditary polyneuropathy.

When an asymptomatic patient goes for a routine eye examination, the ophthalmologist may discover optic disc edema, ptosis, anisocoria, or a Hollenhorst plaque in a retinal blood vessel.

DISCOVERY BY TESTS DONE FOR OTHER REASONS

Automobile accidents and other forms of trauma often lead to brain computed tomography (CT) or magnetic resonance imaging (MRI) scans. These scans occasionally reveal chronic asymptomatic abnormalities. Congenital disorders, such as agenesis of the corpus callosum, need not be pursued. On the other hand, discovery of an asymptomatic glioma or pituitary adenoma will require monitoring and management decisions. Most asymptomatic

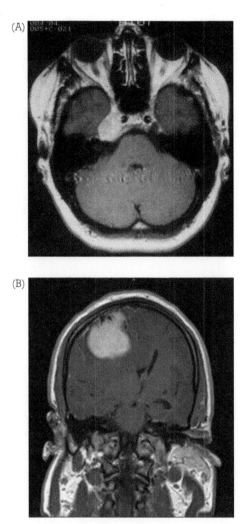

Figure 8.1 Two patients with asymptomatic meningiomas discovered at routine eye examination.

meningiomas simply can be monitored with sequential scans (Figure 8.1).[1] Other asymptomatic tumors can be discovered (Figure 8.2). Scans can also reveal asymptomatic demyelinative disease (Figure 8.3).[2] Patients with such findings will require careful neurological history, examination, and monitoring. Most commonly discovered by scan are various forms of cerebrovascular disease. Old cerebral infarcts, hemorrhages, microhemorrhages, subdural hematomas, arterial stenoses, aneurysms, and vascular malformations can be unexpectedly found. The details in each case will determine what management is appropriate.

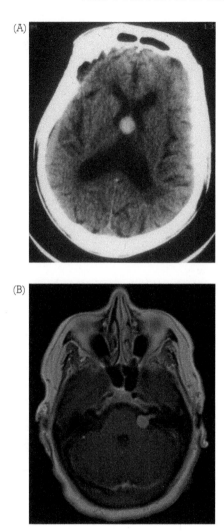

Figure 8.2 Asymptomatic tumors. (A) An asymptomatic colloid cyst of the third ventricle. (B) An asymptomatic acoustic neuroma.

Nerve conduction and electromyography can show asymptomatic abnormalities. Nearly 15% of patients have fibrillations and positive sharp waves on needle examinations of the lumbosacral paraspinal muscles. The prevalence is higher in older patients. Thus, one must be cautious in using spontaneous activity seen in lumbosacral paraspinal muscles to support the diagnosis of radiculopathy as the cause for leg pain.[3] On nerve conduction, one may also find asymptomatic disease like polyneuropathy, mononeuropathies, or Eaton-Lambert myasthenic syndrome.

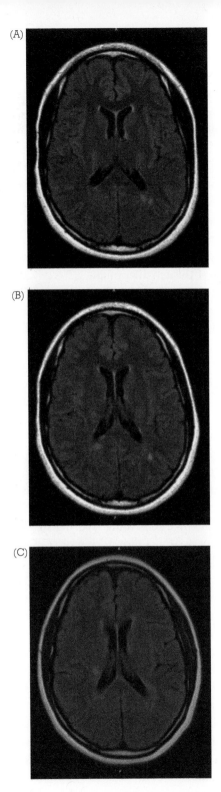

Figure 8.3 Sequential scans done on a patient for sinus problems. Only at the time of the third scan, years after the first scan, was the patient symptomatic from multiple sclerosis. The earlier scans show the lesions accumulating.

PURPOSEFUL SEARCH

One may consider searching for familial disease in asymptomatic patients at risk. Various methods have been tried to detect presymptomatic Huntington disease, but test results can be indeterminate. Patients who choose to determine their gene carrier status may not cope well with the result. In adrenoleukodystrophy MRI brain scans, neuropsychological tests, and other methods have been used to seek an early diagnosis in asymptomatic patients at risk. When there emerges an effective therapy for presymptomatic disease, the search for asymptomatic disease will become standard practice. Should one order an MRI scan on the identical twin of a multiple sclerosis patient? We await data to help us with such dilemmas.

Before initiating anticoagulant therapy for atrial fibrillation, the neurologist commonly orders a scan to check for asymptomatic hemorrhagic transformation of an embolic brain infarct.[4] Often one delays anticoagulation for some days if fresh bleeding is discovered. Likewise, a scan following thrombolytic therapy for stroke can reveal asymptomatic hemorrhagic transformation of the infarction. Whether such findings affect patient management depends on the specifics of each case. (I was interested to learn that, for research purposes, symptomatic hemorrhagic transformation has been categorized as asymptomatic unless the associated symptoms have increased the National Institute of Health [NIH] Stroke Scale greater than 3 points; Amie Hsia, MD, in conversation, 2016).

Arterial imaging is often advocated for endocarditis patients with or without stroke. When an asymptomatic mycotic aneurysm is discovered, experts differ in their recommendations, some favoring surgery, some endovascular intervention, and others simple monitoring of the aneurysm during antibiotic therapy.

Screening for berry aneurysm is discussed in two kinds of patients. First, there are individuals who have a strong family history of berry aneurysm. Second, there are those with autosomal dominant polycystic kidney disease. In patients with a history of familial aneurysm (at least two affected first-degree relatives), close to 30% may harbor an intracranial aneurysm.[5] Whereas screening such patients may be helpful, screening of relatives of a patient with sporadic aneurysmal subarachnoid hemorrhage is not recommended.[6] In autosomal dominant polycystic kidney disease there is an increased risk of berry aneurysm. However, if there has been no diagnosis of berry aneurysm in a family member, screening is not useful. When the patient has the kidney disease and a family history of aneurysm, the advantages and disadvantages of screening should be discussed with the patient.[7]

MAJOR TOPICS

In neurologic practice, asymptomatic lesions have been most discussed in the realm of cerebrovascular disease. Attention has centered on carotid stenosis, berry aneurysm, and arteriovenous malformation.

Once one has discovered an asymptomatic berry aneurysm, the doctor and patient must decide how to use the information (Figure 8.4). All agree that tobacco use and arterial hypertension should be avoided. In addition, one must explain to the patient that whatever symptoms may have led to the scan, they are not related to the aneurysm. The big question is whether to directly treat the aneurysm by clipping at open surgery or by an interventional catheterization method such as coiling. Treatment is motivated by the desire to prevent rupture. However, there is no high-quality evidence to support such treatment of asymptomatic intracranial aneurysms.[8] Aneurysm size is often weighed heavily in decisions about whether one should intervene. Recommendations will evolve as new data are published.

Improved methods of interventional treatment for arteriovenous malformations have emerged in recent decades. Whether or not to utilize such methods in asymptomatic cases has been investigated. [9] Death and stroke were less common in the patients receiving medical therapy than in those receiving combined medical therapy and interventional treatment. Those inclined to interventional treatment point out the imperfections of such data and view the results differently.[10] Data are hard to obtain and interpret because the malformations are heterogeneous.

Of all asymptomatic diseases, carotid stenosis in the neck has attracted the most attention over the past half century. Stenosis may be detected by physical exam (cervical bruit) or carotid ultrasound. The development of endarterectomy led confident vascular surgeons to treat asymptomatic lesions. Years of experience showed the morbidity of the operation to be considerable in community hospitals. Finally, it was proved that endarterectomy was beneficial for severe stenosis when it was performed with the low morbidity rates reported in the investigational setting. Controversy on this subject did not cease. Because intra-arterial catheter-based treatments were shown to match the morbidity and mortality of carotid surgery, some believed that these interventional methods were preferable. Meanwhile, there came improvements in the medical management of hyperlipidemia and other risk factors for stroke. With this medical progress, experts eventually began to question the relevance of older research supporting surgery. Management practice for asymptomatic carotid stenosis varies from one specialty to another.[11] Educating the patient about the ever-changing data and any extant controversy will always be important in deciding whether one should intervene.[12]

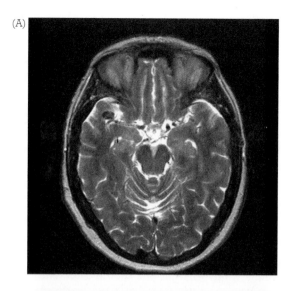

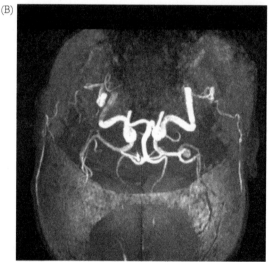

Figure 8.4 Asymptomatic aneurysm. An otolaryngologist ordered brain magnetic resonance imaging for this 60-year-old nurse's complaint of hearing loss. The pictured berry aneurysm (A) was asymptomatic, as were a second berry aneurysm and a small meningioma. After coiling of this aneurysm, she developed aphasia and hemiparesis. After months of recovery, she could walk independently and communicate well but imperfectly. She declined when the surgeon suggested that the second aneurysm be sealed. The patient in (B) reported weakness of one arm. The scan ordered by the internist showed a berry aneurysm. A neurologist determined that the arm weakness was due to a radial neuropathy.

Less controversial is the subject of carotid or vertebral artery occlusion. It is not unusual for one or more of these large vessels to become occluded without symptoms if the collateral circulation is good. With total occlusion, no surgical intervention is possible. The finding of occlusion does indicate the need to pursue and manage atherosclerosis risk factors.

Asymptomatic papilledema is a major topic outside the field of cerebrovascular disease. Brain images exclude tumor as the cause. Typically, such cases are obese young women with idiopathic increased intracranial pressure. Only lumbar puncture can confirm the presence of increased intracranial pressure and exclude chronic meningitis. Occasionally, a lumbar puncture can be avoided. An asymptomatic person may be taking a medicine, such as tetracycline, which can increase intracranial pressure. If there has been no visual field loss, one may be able to discontinue the medicine, monitor the visual fields, and await resolution of the papilledema. When in doubt, one must do the lumbar puncture.

FINAL COMMENTS

1. It is usually clear whether a lesion is asymptomatic or symptomatic. There are exceptions. I remember one patient with seizures that were, in the end, proved to be nonepileptic. When the patient underwent a brain MRI, a glioma was discovered. It was never clear whether the glioma had been asymptomatic, unrelated to the "seizures," or whether it had been symptomatic, causing personality and behavioral changes with consequent nonepileptic spells.
2. When one considers treating asymptomatic disease, it has been said, "The question before any intervention is not how poor the prognosis is without it, but how much better it is with it."[13]

REFERENCES

1. Go RS, Taylor B V, Kimmel DW. The natural history of asymptomatic meningiomas in Olmsted County, Minnesota. *Neurology*. 1998;51(6):1718–1720.
2. Lebrun C, Bensa C, Debouverie M, Wiertlevski S, Brassat D, de Seze J, Rumbach L, et al. Association between clinical conversion to multiple sclerosis in radiologically isolated syndrome and magnetic resonance imaging, cerebrospinal fluid, and visual evoked potential: follow-up of 70 patients. *Arch Neurol*. 2009;66(7):841–846.
3. Dale ES, Mar EY, Bugola MR, Teraoka JK. The prevalence of lumbar paraspinal spontaneous activity in asymptomatic subjects. *Muscle Nerve*. 1996;19(3):350–354.

4. Laureno R, shields RW Jr., Narayan R. The diagnosis and management of cerebral embolism and hemorrhagic infarction with sequential computerized cranial tomography. *Brain.* 1987;110:93–105.

5. Alberts MJ, Quinones A, Graffagnino C, Friedman A, Roses AD. Risk of intracranial aneurysms in families with subarachnoid hemorrhage. *Can J Neurol Sci.* 1995;22(2):121–125.

6. Ronkainen A, Miettinen H, Karkola K, Papinaho S, Vanninen R, Puranen M, Hernesniemi J. Risk of harboring an unruptured intracranial aneurysm. *Stroke.* 1998;29(2):359–362.

7. Pirson Y, Chauveau D, Torres V. Management of cerebral aneurysms in autosomal dominant polycystic kidney disease. *J Am Soc Nephrol.* 2002;13(1):269–276.

8. Mayer TE. The unruptured intracranial aneurysm treatment score: a multidisciplinary consensus. *Neurology.* 2016;86(8):792–793.

9. Mohr JP, Parides MK, Stapf C, Moquete E, Moy CS, Overbey JR, Al-Shahi Salman R, et al. Medical management with or without interventional therapy for unruptured brain arteriovenous malformations (ARUBA): a multicentre, non-blinded, randomised trial. *Lancet (London, England).* 2014;383(9917):614–621.

10. Day AL, Dannenbaum M, Jung S. A randomized trial of unruptured brain arteriovenous malformations trial: an editorial review. *Stroke.* 2014;45(10):3147–3148.

11. Schrooten M, Fourneau I, Thijs V, Verhamme P, Nevelsteen A. Does medical specialty influence the treatment of asymptomatic carotid stenosis? A Belgian multidisciplinary survey. *J Cardiovasc Surg (Torino).* 2011;52(2):153–157.

12. Spence JD, Naylor AR. Endarterectomy, stenting, or neither for asymptomatic carotid-artery stenosis. *N Engl J Med.* 2016;374(11):1087–1088.

13. Prasad V. An unmeasured harm of screening. *Arch Intern Med.* 2012;172 (19):1442–1443.

PART THREE

Perspectives on Neurology

9

Terminology

Terms from classical languages came to medicine in waves. Some originated in ancient times, some developed when Latin was the language of scholars in the Renaissance and during the Scientific Revolution, and some emerged in modern times. The resulting language of medicine is mainly a Latinized Greek. By and large, the vocabulary is Greek and the structure is Latin. The two main roots of our medical terminology have given us some duplicate terms. "Pituitary" is Latin for phlegm; "hypophysis" is Greek for undergrowth. "Cerebrum" is purely Latin, whereas "encephalon" is Greek.

For prefixes and suffixes, Greek dominates. The Greek prefix, "a," means without. We use it every day in "alexia," "aphasia," and "abulia," to name a few. The prefix "para" means abnormal. The term for vision in Greek is "opsia" or "opia." Both are quoted in an 1888 book on the language of medicine. Most derivative terms consistently employ one form of the suffix or the other (e.g., micr*opsia* on one hand and my*opia* on the other).[1] However, in one situation, either form can be used. Hemianopsia and hemianopia are interchangeable. Some doctors strongly prefer one suffix and some the other (Figures 9.1–9.4).

Old medical terms were more likely to be purely Greek or Latin in origin. In the United States, in particular, there had been, by the 19th century, a decline in knowledge of classical languages, and doctors mixed the languages when creating medical terms. Thus, quadriplegia has become more popular in America than the purely Greek tetraplegia. Myasthenia (Greek) gravis (Latin) is another hybrid term. In the second half of the 20th century, new terms continued to violate linguistic purity: central pontine (Latin) myelinolysis (Greek) is an example. Many hybrid terms prevail despite the objections of pedants.

AJO®
AMERICAN JOURNAL OF OPHTHALMOLOGY®
MONTHLY SINCE 1884

SUITE 1415   435 N. MICHIGAN AVENUE   CHICAGO, IL 60611   (312) 787-3853   FAX (312) 787-5186

Frank W. Newell, M.D., Publisher and Editor-in-Chief
Mary L. Borysewicz, Executive Managing Editor

16 July 1991

Jonathan C. Horton, M.D.
Neuro-Ophthalmology Unit
U-125 University of California
San Francisco, CA 94143-0350

Dear Dr. Horton:

Your telephone call concerning the word "hemianopsia"
perplexed us. Although you stated that you had used the word
"hemianopia" in The Journal in previous years, we could not
find your name among our authors. Similarly, your statement
that the word in the 1990 Stedman's Medical Dictionary was
outdated concerned us.

As far as I can determine, "opia" refers to the eye and is
used in words such as "myopia." "Opsia" refers to vision and
is used in words such as "hemianopsia." The Index Medicus,
which lists titles, uses the word "hemianopsia" in its key word
index, with no reference to hemianopia.

I am perplexed at your insistence on the use of
hemianopia. The AMA journals do not use it and I can find no
standard reference that uses it. Please write and tell the
basis of preference.

Sincerely yours,

Frank W. Newell, M.D.

cc: Marvin Alper, M.D.
     Beth Foor, Manuscript Editor

encl.
K525
FWN/mm

Figure 9.1 Letters disagreeing about terminology should be read sequentially from Figures 9.1 through 9.4. In this first letter, the journal editor replies to a telephone call from an author of a submitted article. (Provided by Jonathan Horton, MD.)

Words evolve in meaning. For the ancients, the "neuro" root was used for both nerves and tendons. Thomas Willis coined the term "neurologie" to refer to the anatomy of cranial, spinal, and autonomic nerves.[2] Gradually, however, the word came to its current meaning: the study or knowledge of the peripheral and central nervous systems. There are many other examples of

UNIVERSITY OF CALIFORNIA, SAN FRANCISCO

BERKELEY · DAVIS · IRVINE · LOS ANGELES · RIVERSIDE · SAN DIEGO · SAN FRANCISCO   SANTA BARBARA · SANTA CRUZ

DEPARTMENT OF NEUROLOGICAL SURGERY
NEURO-OPHTHALMOLOGY UNIT   SAN FRANCISCO, CALIFORNIA 94143
126 UC HOSPITAL
(415) 476-1130   22 July 1991

Frank W. Newell MD
American Journal of Ophthalmology
435 N. Michigan Avenue, Suite 1415
Chicago, Illinois 60611

Dear Dr. Newell,

Thank you for your letter of 16 July 1991 concerning the word "hemianop[s]ia.

I am not a Greek scholar, but I believe that "opia" and "opsia" are both derived from the Greek word "ops", meaning eye or vision. From a historical perspective, ophthalmologists have traditionally used the term "hemianopsia", and your defense of this term is legitimate and correct. On the other hand, "homonymous hemianopsia" catches in the mouth of many physicians and I think that we have an obligation to undertake any effort that we can to ease oral communication. Dropping the "s" does make the word slide out a bit easier.

Perhaps for this reason, a strong trend has developed in favor of "hemianopia", rather than "hemianopsia". For example, the 3d edition of Walsh & Hoyt's Clinical Neuro-Ophthalmology used "hemianopsia" exclusively. However, with the 4th edition, Dr. Neil Miller, with the full agreement of Dr. William Hoyt, has switched completely to "hemianopia", and you will not so much as find "hemianopsia" in the textbook index.

In your letter you stated that the AMA journals do not use hemianopia. In the June 1991 issue of the Archives of Ophthalmology, Dr. Hoyt and I published an article on the representation of the visual field in human striate cortex and we used the word "hemianopia" throughout. I have reviewed the last two years of the Archives of Ophthalmology and have found both "hemianopia" and "hemianopsia". I presume the matter has been left to the preference of the author. It is worth noting that "hemianopia" was used much more often than "hemianopsia".

I have the 22d edition of Stedman's Medical Dictionary. I purchased it when I decided to become a doctor upon my graduation from high school in 1972. Under "hemianopia" it simply provides the entry: "hemianopsia". Under "hemianopsia" it supplies the actual definition of the term. This arrangement implies that "hemianopsia" is the preferred usage. I think this edition of Stedman's is outdated in this respect, inasmuch as use of "hemianopia" has truly gained ascendency.

Figure 9.2 The author of the article replies to the editor. (Provided by Jonathan Horton, MD.)

transformation of word meaning. The word "infarction" (derived from the Latin term for "stuffed") was originally applied to cerebral hemorrhage. Over time, it became applied to brain necrosis due to an area of focal ischemia. "Nystagmus" (derived from the Greek term for nodding or drowsiness) is now used for the rhythmic involuntary movements of the eyes. "Inflammation"

Finally, I apologize for the misunderstanding when I said to Ms. Foor that "we've used hemianopia before in the Journal". By "we", I meant the Neuro-Ophthalmology Unit at UCSF which I joined last year. I enclose an article from our Unit published a few years ago in the AJO by Drs. Tychsen & Hoyt, with use of "hemianopia".

I hope these comments shed some light on my rather dogged efforts to persuade you to allow us to use "hemianopia" in our upcoming article.

Sincerely,

Jonathan Horton

Jonathan C. Horton MD PhD

Enclosure

CC: Ms Beth Foor, Manuscript Editor
      Marvin Alper MD

Figure 9.2 Continued

originally indicated a clinical condition and later a microscopic one. Today, many think of it as a biochemical response. The word "dystonia" has been used variously. Oppenheim was an early user of the term; he applied it to a specific disease. Wilson used it for any change in muscle tone, and Denny Brown applied it to the increased tone of a spastic hemiparesis and other phenomena. Currently, "dystonia" refers to an involuntary posture which is, for a time, sustained rather than constantly changing, like the related phenomena

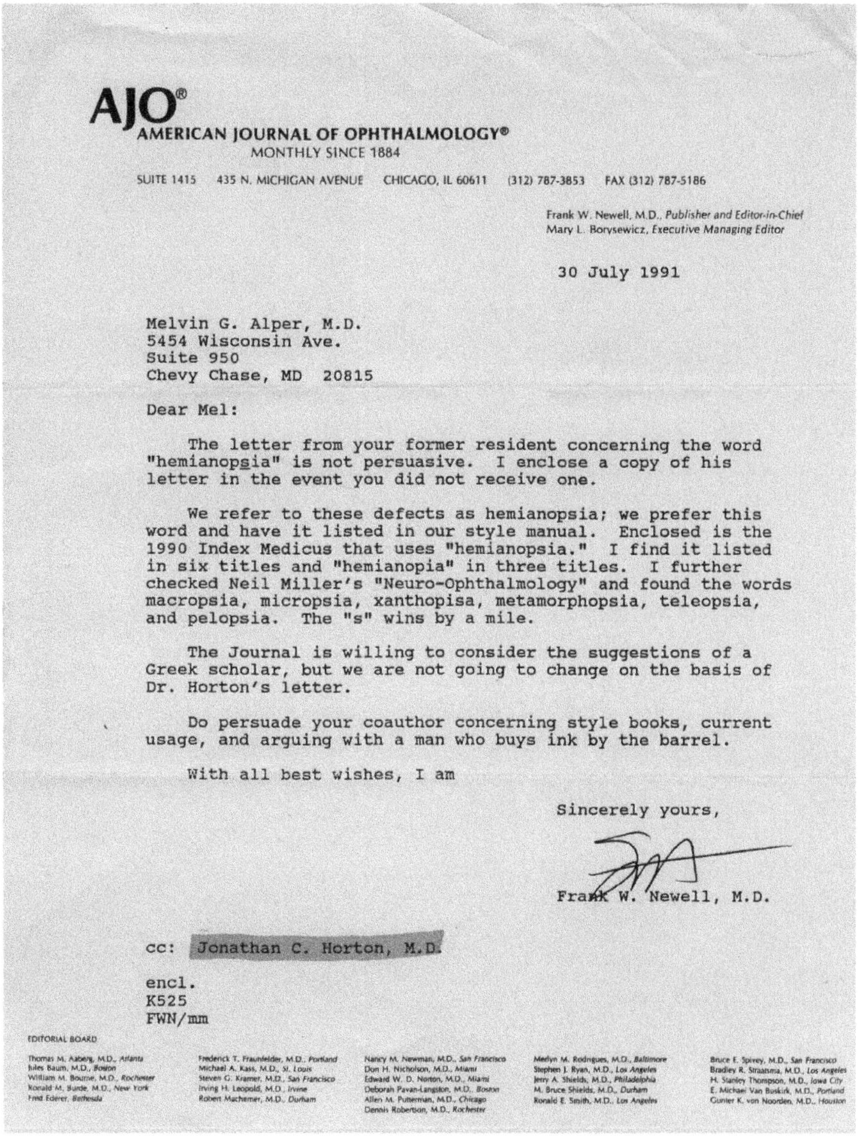

AJO®
AMERICAN JOURNAL OF OPHTHALMOLOGY®
MONTHLY SINCE 1884

SUITE 1415   435 N. MICHIGAN AVENUE   CHICAGO, IL 60611   (312) 787-3853   FAX (312) 787-5186

Frank W. Newell, M.D., *Publisher and Editor-in-Chief*
Mary L. Borysewicz, *Executive Managing Editor*

30 July 1991

Melvin G. Alper, M.D.
5454 Wisconsin Ave.
Suite 950
Chevy Chase, MD 20815

Dear Mel:

   The letter from your former resident concerning the word
"hemianopsia" is not persuasive. I enclose a copy of his
letter in the event you did not receive one.

   We refer to these defects as hemianopsia; we prefer this
word and have it listed in our style manual. Enclosed is the
1990 Index Medicus that uses "hemianopsia." I find it listed
in six titles and "hemianopia" in three titles. I further
checked Neil Miller's "Neuro-Ophthalmology" and found the words
macropsia, micropsia, xanthopisa, metamorphopsia, teleopsia,
and pelopsia. The "s" wins by a mile.

   The Journal is willing to consider the suggestions of a
Greek scholar, but we are not going to change on the basis of
Dr. Horton's letter.

   Do persuade your coauthor concerning style books, current
usage, and arguing with a man who buys ink by the barrel.

   With all best wishes, I am

                                         Sincerely yours,

                                         Frank W. Newell, M.D.

cc: Jonathan C. Horton, M.D.

encl.
K525
FWN/mm

Figure 9.3 The editor responds to a co-author. (Provided by Jonathan Horton, MD.)

of chorea and athetosis. It has been said that words are like territories—they
can be taken over.

   Terms must compete for dominance or even survival in the medical literature. Tetanus had been known to Pliny. Two millennia after his time, another
less severe form of involuntary muscle contractions was recognized. Trousseau
suggested the term "tetanilla" (little tetanus) to distinguish this condition

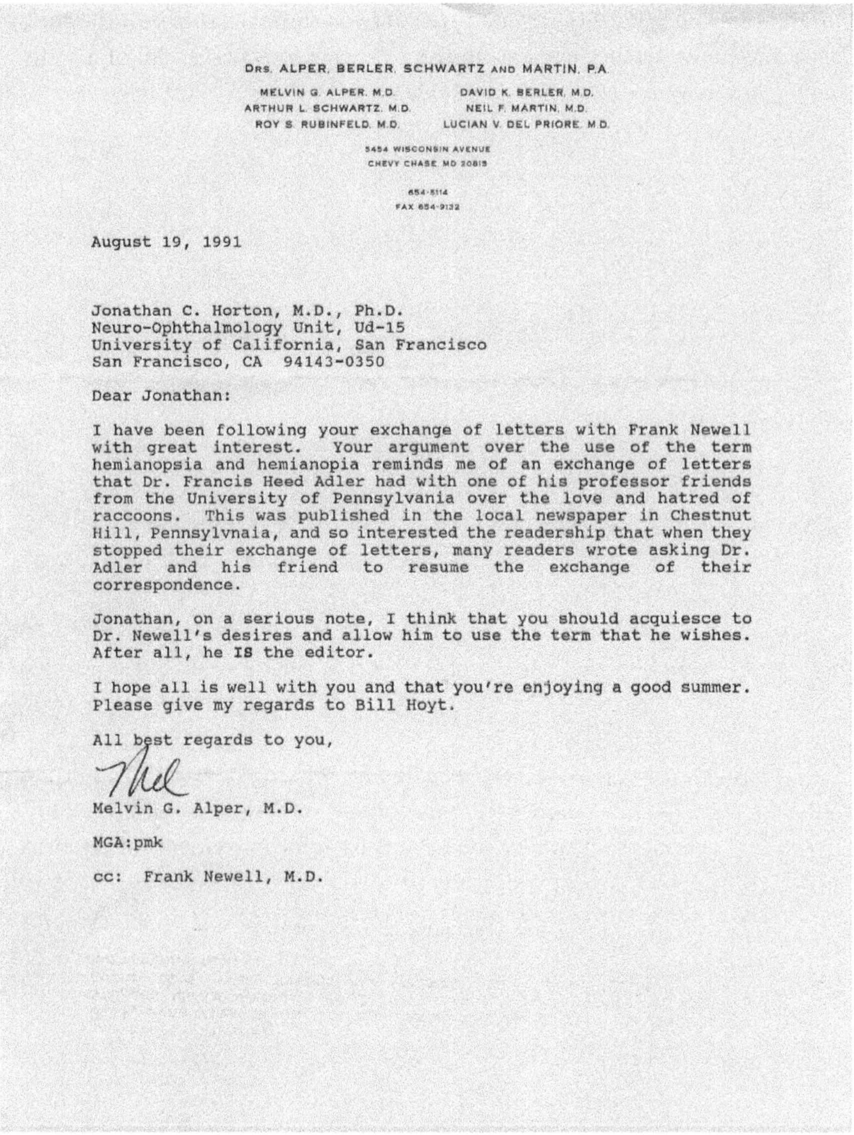

DRS. ALPER, BERLER, SCHWARTZ AND MARTIN, P.A.

MELVIN G. ALPER, M.D.   DAVID K. BERLER, M.D.
ARTHUR L. SCHWARTZ, M.D.   NEIL F. MARTIN, M.D.
ROY S. RUBINFELD, M.D.   LUCIAN V. DEL PRIORE, M.D.

5454 WISCONSIN AVENUE
CHEVY CHASE, MD 20815

654-5114
FAX 654-9132

August 19, 1991

Jonathan C. Horton, M.D., Ph.D.
Neuro-Ophthalmology Unit, Ud-15
University of California, San Francisco
San Francisco, CA 94143-0350

Dear Jonathan:

I have been following your exchange of letters with Frank Newell
with great interest. Your argument over the use of the term
hemianopsia and hemianopia reminds me of an exchange of letters
that Dr. Francis Heed Adler had with one of his professor friends
from the University of Pennsylvania over the love and hatred of
raccoons. This was published in the local newspaper in Chestnut
Hill, Pennsylvnaia, and so interested the readership that when they
stopped their exchange of letters, many readers wrote asking Dr.
Adler and his friend to resume the exchange of their
correspondence.

Jonathan, on a serious note, I think that you should acquiesce to
Dr. Newell's desires and allow him to use the term that he wishes.
After all, he IS the editor.

I hope all is well with you and that you're enjoying a good summer.
Please give my regards to Bill Hoyt.

All best regards to you,

Melvin G. Alper, M.D.

MGA:pmk

cc: Frank Newell, M.D.

Figure 9.4 The co-author writes to the first author. (Provided by Jonathan Horton, MD.)

from lockjaw. The term tètanie, however, has prevailed. Perhaps, its being one syllable shorter has contributed to "tetany's" success.

Such competition between words continues. Border zone infarctions are described as "borderland," "end zone," "boundary zone," "terminal zone," and "watershed." Bladin et al. explain that the "border zone" is a proper description of infarction occurring at the overlap area of two arterial territories.[3] They also explain that a "watershed" relates to the drainage, not perfusion, of a water system. They nevertheless seem comfortable with the current preference for the incorrect term "watershed."

There have been many competing terms for giant cell arteritis. Horton's disease seems to have lost out. Granulomatous arteritis and cranial arteritis are seldom heard, whereas giant cell arteritis (emphasizing only one feature of the microscopic pathology) and temporal arteritis (emphasizing a typically involved artery) are both used with some frequency.

Common syncope, which is a neurally mediated reflex, has had many names. Thomas Lewis applied the term "vaso-vagal" to this condition. He used the term to indicate that the blood pressure drop was due to *vaso*dilatation and that the bradycardia was *vagal*ly mediated. Vasodepressor syncope was a synonym. A new term, "neurocardiogenic syncope," appeared in 1991. This term focuses attention on the role of afferents from the heart in the genesis of the faint. This term does not indicate the fundamental role of bradycardia and vasodilatation in the syncopal event. Nevertheless, the new name was "consecrated by an adulatory three-page editorial" in the *New England Journal of Medicine*.[4] Although this polysyllabic, anointed term seems to be dominating, "vaso-vagal" has not yet disappeared from the clinical lexicon.

Exceptionally, a word is successful when it is used for a wide variety of conditions that have no anatomic, physiologic, or etiologic commonality. "Myoclonus" is the best example. The term is used for movements of cerebral, cerebellar, brainstem, and spinal origin. The movements can be localized or generalized. Somehow, it has proved useful to retain this wide-net word for these various rapid movements.

Over time, the origins of a term can be forgotten. Where, for example, did the term "mycotic aneurysm" originate? One of the old names for endocarditis was mycosis endocardii because fungating vegetations were present on the cardiac valves. The occurrence of cerebral aneurysm, in the setting of these valvular lesions, led to the term "mycotic aneurysm." The word indicates the gross appearance of the heart finding. It has nothing to do with infection by a fungus.[5]

Doctors can define and use a term very differently. In one department at Massachusetts General Hospital, leading figures could not agree. Raymond Adams used the term "delirium" to indicate a hyperalert state of total disorientation and autonomic hyperactivity. C. Miller Fisher, his colleague, used the word in a more general sense to indicate a confusional state with or without obtundation. There continues to be a split in the medical community over appropriate usage of this term.

Simultaneously, two medical specialties may use different words for one clinical disorder. Nephrologists use the term "rhabdomyolysis," focusing attention on muscle injury. On the other hand, many neurologists use the word "myoglobinuria," emphasizing the urinary findings.[6] There are difficulties with both terms. Hence, Raymond Adams and Maurice Victor preferred the term "pan-necrotizing myopathy" for this disorder. Another example is the term "benediction hand." It refers to a pathologic positioning of the fingers resembling that assumed by a pope making a blessing (i.e., "the ring and small fingers are flexed and the index and middle fingers are not").[7] Neurologists use the term for the finger positioning seen when a patient with a high median neuropathy attempts to make a fist. Internists and orthopedists use the term to refer to the claw deformity of distal ulnar neuropathy.

The term "cerebral palsy" is problematic in that the affected patients share no common etiology or pathology. I was taught that "cerebral palsy" was a lay term, that it did not distinguish cerebral infarction from kernicterus or subependymal hemorrhage. In the same vein, Karin Nelson remembers being taught that some of the affected patients had problems that were neither cerebral nor palsy (Karin Nelson, MD, in conversation, 2016). She considers the common denominator for cerebral palsy patients to be a disorder of movement. The term is "general enough to indicate that the brain was not made right or that it was damaged early on" (Karin Nelson, MD, in conversation, 2016). It appears that "cerebral palsy" remains a useful category for this heterogeneous group of patients.[8]

Some appealing terms are widely misused. The term "tardy ulnar palsy" was developed for a traumatic ulnar neuropathy at a specific location. Doctors, assuming that there had been unrecognized prior trauma, began to use it for any ulnar neuropathy at the elbow. Likewise "cubital tunnel syndrome" designated compression of the nerve by the humeroulnar aponeurotic arcade. This term also degenerated into a generic term for any ulnar neuropathy at the elbow. The misuse of these perfectly good terms resulted from a lack of physician knowledge. Many neurologists did not understand the detailed anatomy and variability of the ulnar nerve's course at the elbow. Thus they could appreciate neither the vulnerability of the nerve at different sites in the elbow region nor the nontraumatic etiologies of ulnar neuropathy at the elbow.[9]

Some frequently used terms are fundamentally mistaken. One often hears of the "empty sella." Incompetence of the diaphragm of the sella turcica is a normal anatomical variant. It allows the subarachnoid space to work its way into the sella turcica. The cerebrospinal fluid fills the sella turcica, and its pounding pressure flattens the pituitary. On images, the sella turcica is "empty" only in the sense that a normally plump pituitary is not seen. The worst usage is the term "empty sella syndrome" because there is no consistent syndrome associated with this normal anatomical variant. In most instances, patients are asymptomatic.

Particularly puzzling is the persistence of the misnomer "bovine aortic arch." There is a common anatomical variant in which the left common carotid artery and the innominate artery do not arise individually from the aortic arch. Instead, they arise from a common origin. For some reason, this configuration has been referred to as a "bovine aortic arch," although it is never seen in cattle.[10]

Terms can mislead a doctor's thinking. Aggressive treatment of high blood pressure can worsen the stroke in patients with acute brain infarction. This observation led to the very good recommendation that hypertension be tolerated or permitted in acute stroke management. Thus emerged the peculiar term "permissive hypertension," which caught on in the general medical community. Knowing the concept and the term, some doctors began to withhold blood pressure medicines from normotensive stroke patients who had been taking them prior to their strokes. Permitting hypertension in such cases really amounted to producing hypertension, which had never been recommended. Sometimes the resulting hypertension can be severe. The catchy term had affected the practice and thinking of some doctors in a way that had not been intended.

Terms are sometimes viewed as being intentionally misleading. The American research enterprise, the Human Genome Project, is a "multiply misleading" term because there is no one human genome and no one project.[11] Studying human genetic variation can go on indefinitely, and thus "the project" can be extended and funded with "no foreseeable terminus." Terming it accurately as "the genome business" would not have engendered public or legislative support.[11] Another example is the term, "sedation for the imminently dying." This term is used by palliative care specialists. Neurologists have explored the ethics of the practice without questioning the term itself.[12] Rady and Verheijde[13] have suggested that sedation for very ill persons should be termed "continuous deep sedation until death." Those who call it "sedation for the imminently dying," they state, disguise the reality that such sedation is a form of physician-assisted death.

RENAMING

With scientific advance, renaming is important and appropriate. Infantile paralysis was a good name for a newly described clinical entity. A century was required for recognition that the pathology is an inflammatory process in the gray matter of the spinal cord and that the disease can affect older children and adults. Hence, the disease was renamed "poliomyelitis." This was progress.

Another example, "otitic hydrocephalus," was the term for the papilledema and headache consequent to inner ear infection. When it was realized that there was no hydrocephalus in such cases, the term pseudotumor cerebri emerged. The idea was that papilledema makes one worry about a tumor, but there is no tumor. (In our era, most cases of this syndrome are not related to ear infection.) Because pseudotumor was basically a problem with increased intracranial pressure, the term benign (i.e., not a tumor) intracranial hypertension was advanced. However, the condition was not benign when it caused blindness. Hence, the term "idiopathic intracranial hypertension" was touted. Of course, not all cases were idiopathic. Currently, some authors have returned to using pseudotumor, either idiopathic pseudotumor cerebri or pseudotumor cerebri syndrome due to a specified cause. Others argue that it is more appropriate to name something for what it is rather than for what it is not. Avoiding the prefix "pseudo," Wall and Corbett prefer the term idiopathic intracranial hypertension when the cause is unknown. When the cause is known, they specify it: for example, intracranial hypertension due to sagittal sinus thrombosis or intracranial hypertension due to vitamin A toxicity.[14]

Terms are changed for social and political reasons. For example "mental retardation" was an enlightened term chosen to replace words like "feeble mindedness" and "mental subnormality," which some considered pejorative. With time "mental retardation" itself came to carry a negative connotation to the lay person. Hence the word "developmental delay" became preferred. These trends have been associated with changes in the title of a medical journal aimed to advance the study of these conditions. There was no negative connotation intended when the *American Journal of Mental Deficiency* was founded in 1895. The name was changed to the *American Journal of Mental Retardation* in 1987, evidently to avoid the perception of disrespect to the patients. Because "mental retardation" also came to be deemed derogatory, there was again renaming. As of 2009, it became the *American Journal of Intellectual and Developmental Disabilities*. In 2010, an act of congress (Rosa's Law) replaced any prior legislative reference to "mental retardation" not with "developmental delay" but with "intellectual disability." Perhaps, in time, the term "disability" will be considered pejorative and there will be demands for further change. The freshness of a new term temporarily relieves the perceived stigma of an old one.

The International League Against Epilepsy felt the need to change its name to the International League for Epilepsy. Presumably the change was intended to sound more supportive of patients and families. Of course, the original purpose of the League and its original name were selected with the best of intentions. Name change can give a feeling of accomplishment when the change has accomplished nothing. Along with the change in organizational name there is a trend toward avoidance of the word "epileptic." Rather than have the disease define the person, some doctors are emphasizing that the person has a disease. Hence the term "people with epilepsy" is being used by some experts in preference to "epileptics."[15]

Driven by concerns about opprobrium and accuracy, the term for hysterical seizures has successively been changed to pseudoseizures, psychogenic seizures, nonepileptic seizures, and nonepileptic behavioral episodes. "Hysterical" was understood to connote an emotional female and was considered pejorative. The term "pseudo" was deemed disrespectful to the patient because it implied deceit. We do not understand how the psyche might cause such episodes. Thus "psychogenic" was abandoned and "nonepileptic seizure" was adopted. Soon, however, some doctors suggested that, if such events were not truly seizures, they should not be called seizures. They renamed them "nonepileptic behavioral episodes." Many of these terms continue to be used.

When Plum and colleagues were studying coma patients, they frequently had to counsel families about prognosis. A relative would commonly worry that the patient would end up as a "vegetable." Following the lead of these lay persons, Plum and Jennett proposed the term "vegetative state." This term referred to patients who, emerging from coma, opened their eyes, resumed sleep–wake cycles, but remained unresponsive and unaware. This nonpejorative term was widely used for half a century. Now, perceiving the term disrespectful, authors have proposed an alternative, "unresponsive wakefulness syndrome." Again opprobrium, it has been explained, was perceived where there was none intended.[16]

In a push for the nonstigmatizing, perfect term, we often end up with a very nonspecific word. The term "nonepileptic behavioral episode" could apply to a temper tantrum. "Intellectual disability" could include dyslexia and dementia as well as mental retardation, the term it was intended to replace. It is hard to see any medical value in the use of such vague terms as "intellectual disability" and "nonepileptic behavioral episodes."

Avoidance of opprobrium is not the only reason for the adoption of overly inclusive terms. "Striatonigral degeneration" did not indicate the associated degeneration of other neural systems, especially autonomic neurons. Hence, a new name was proposed and popularized. This umbrella term, "multiple system atrophy," is far from ideal. It is applied to a very heterogeneous group of patients. Furthermore, there are many other diseases in which multiple systems degenerate.

The variability of intracranial arteries can lead to confusion in naming. The anterior cerebellum is typically supplied by the anterior inferior cerebellar artery (AICA), which arises from the basilar artery. In some patients, a similar artery arises from the vertebral artery rather than from the basilar artery. About such a case, the neurosurgeon may say that, "the AICA arises from the vertebral artery." A purist angiographer may disagree, explaining that, by definition, the AICA is an artery that comes off the basilar artery and supplies the anterior cerebellum. In other words it should only be called AICA when it arises from the basilar artery. (William Bank, M.D., in conversation, 2013).

Investigation of the genetics of human disease has led to challenges to traditional nomenclature. Since there is no one gene for Parkinson disease, some have proposed an alternate term, Parkinson diseases. Only if individual genetic causes of these diseases were proved to have different therapies or prognoses would such a term be appropriate. Because "ataxia telangiectasia" can occur with neither ataxia nor telangiectasia, some would prefer a more encompassing genetic term for the disease. Because not all patients with Huntington's chorea have the movement disorder, the term Huntington disease has been suggested as preferable. To head in the direction of these suggested changes would dissociate our terms from any clinical aspect.

EPONYMS[17]

There are no simple rules, which determine whether or when a medical eponym will be accepted. The publication that leads to an eponym need not be long. Trömner's article of 39 lines led to his eponym. One need not be famous to gain an eponym. The line of Gennari is named for the medical student who found it. Jendrassik was an internal medicine resident when he described his maneuver. Centuries may pass before one's name becomes applied: Sydenham's St. Vitus dance was not called Sydenham's chorea until 200 years after his description.

An eponym does not always refer to a doctor. Rarely a disease or pathogen is named for a patient, such as Hartnup or John Cunningham (JC virus of progressive multifocal leukoencephalopathy). "Lou Gehrig's disease," named for an American baseball player, was once a lay term for amyotrophic lateral sclerosis. Now it can be seen in the titles of scientific articles. Sometimes an eponym is unrelated to a doctor or a patient. Münchausen syndrome is named for a real baron who traveled widely and told fantastic tales. The name of this storyteller became applied when an observer of Münchausen patients was reminded of him.

Applying one's own name to something is seldom successful. Henry Head described areas of the body surface to which various visceral pains may refer. Although he called these "Head's areas," the term did not catch on. Kernig was more successful when he named his sign for himself.

Some names honor doctors who never wrote a word about the subjects of their eponyms. Hoffmann's reflex was described by Hans Curschmann, who had worked as a resident under Hoffmann. In a case report, he placed a footnote calling it "Hoffmann's phenomenon (not published)." Likewise one of Lasègue's students (J. J. Forst) wrote about the sign to which Lasègue had drawn his attention. Lasègue had never written about it.

The prevailing idea is that a structure or phenomenon should be named for the person or persons who first described and best established an entity. The situation is clearest when one person first describes, best describes, and repeatedly describes something in widely read and respected medical journals. Von Economo wrote 27 papers and a book on encephalitis lethargica. It is clearly appropriate that his clinicopathologic studies be remembered by the term Von Economo's encephalitis. Nikolaus Friedreich was clearly the first to describe his ataxia. For Bell's phenomenon, Bell's priority is unchallenged.

However, priority alone seldom determines the eponym. Duchenne was rewarded with an eponym for a detailed but purely clinical description of his dystrophy. History has neglected Meryon's prior report, which had recognized the disease as familial, had shown muscle pathology in drawings, and had correctly argued that dystrophy was a primary muscle disease. Fairness would dictate a hyphenated eponym recognizing both men.

Often there are good reasons for the eponyms going to someone other than those who made the fist description. Clearly, facial palsy had been described before the work of Charles Bell. However, he was the first to understand the nature of the condition. Parkinson credited others with priority in describing paralysis agitans. However, his description of the distinctive syndrome was such that Charcot termed it "la Maladie de Parkinson." The circle of arterial anastomoses at the base of the brain had been described earlier by Fallopio and others, but it was Willis who recognized the importance of this anatomic arrangement. Therefore, Haller referred to it as the "circle of Willis." Likewise, Gowers was not the first to describe his sign; he knew that Duchenne had drawn attention to it. However, Gowers was the first to give a complete description of it. Likewise well-deserved is the eponym "Wallenberg syndrome." There had been an earlier account of the clinical syndrome, but it was Wallenberg who clarified it. In a series of articles, he predicted the location of the lesion and later proved it at autopsy. Similarly, Wilson was not the first to describe a case of what he called progressive lenticular degeneration (Wilson disease). However, he was the one who published a series of cases with autopsy documentation of the brain and liver findings. Lhermitte's sign had been described by Pierre Marie and later by Babinski and then by Devic. Lhermitte focused on the sign's occurrence in three cases of multiple sclerosis; its value in diagnosis brought him an eponym.

A structure known in antiquity, when brought to wide attention in recent centuries, has often been named for the modern observer. Monro credits Galen for describing what we call the foramen of Monro. Likewise, Galen wrote of the aqueduct of the midbrain long before Sylvius did. In such cases, it is the rediscovery that has attached a doctor's name to the structure.

Some well-ingrained eponyms are undeserved. Parinaud never clearly described or localized the syndrome that carries his name. In fact, he was not the first to describe it. Many preceded Adie in describing his syndrome, but Adie wrote his piece in the prestigious journal *Brain* and thereby achieved recognition. On the grounds of priority, Bonnet has dismissed the attribution of oculosympathetic paresis to Horner. "It is not possible to tolerate any more that the name of Horner's syndrome is designated to the paralytic syndrome of the cervical sympathetic in the Anglo Saxon literature." He goes on, "The clinical picture that expresses paralyses of the cervical sympathetic should rightfully carry the name of Poufour du Petit."[17]

Until recently, eponyms have been expressed as possessive adjectives (i.e., Parkinson's disease). "Down's syndrome" was an approved term of the World Health Organization in its 1966 document. This group has never reversed its opinion. However, in 1992, Index Medicus changed its listing of this disease from Down's syndrome to Down syndrome. Editorial boards and statements on preferred medical terminology have followed suit. Uniform usage is important mainly to the pedant. If "Bell palsy" does not roll off the tongue as well as "Bell's palsy," why should one avoid the possessive? "A foolish consistency," said Emerson, "is the hobgoblin of little minds."

Eponyms can recall the contribution of more than one doctor. Guillain, Barré, and Strohl worked together on their seminal paper on albuminocytologic dissociation in acute polyneuropathy. Baker used the term Guillain-Barré, leaving off the third author. Likely he was influenced by Guillain and Barré's having written, without Strohl, several subsequent papers on their subject. Perhaps a three-man eponym is more awkward to use than one with fewer names. Nevertheless, Haymaker called the disease Landry-Guillain-Barré syndrome due to the earlier clinical description by Landry. There is more than one way to see history. Surely Landry-Guillain-Barré-Strohl syndrome is too polysyllabic for use on the hospital wards.

Double names do not always indicate that two authors worked together, like Guillain and Barré. Erb wrote an article describing certain palsies of the arm that he attributed to an upper brachial plexus injury. Duchenne had earlier described a similar syndrome in babies without analysis of localization. The two famous neurologists are remembered by Erb-Duchenne palsy despite Danyan having described this condition 20 years before Duchenne.[17] Likewise, Cheyne and Stokes never worked together. Cheyne observed and reported this

respiratory pattern. However, it was Stokes influential book, wherein he attributed the discovery to Cheyne, which drew attention to the disorder of breathing. Somehow we now know it as Cheyne-Stokes respiration.[17]

At times it is unclear whether a term honors a single person or more than one
individual. Ramsay Hunt, Foster Kennedy, and Brown Séquard are eponyms
that sound like they honor two persons, but each term is the name of one doctor. On the other hand, Martin-Gruber anastomosis sounds like one person
when it is spoken. When one is reading, however, the hyphen indicates that the
term commemorates two doctors.

Politics and personal loyalty play a role in eponyms. Spielmeyer gave
precedence to his student by using the term, Creutzfeldt-Jakob disease.
Kirschbaum gave priority to his teacher by referring to Jakob-Creutzfeldt
disease, a more appropriate designation. After the death of Eaton, a clinician, the loyalty of Mayo clinic faculty and electromyographers to Lambert,
the physiologist, and their appreciation of Lambert's contribution led to the
widespread change in usage from Eaton-Lambert syndrome to Lambert-
Eaton syndrome. This eponym reversal has been more successful in the
United States than elsewhere.

A political campaign can be waged to retract an eponym. No one doubted
that Friedreich Wegener's work deserved an eponym. When it was discovered
and publicized in 2011 that Wegener had joined the *Sturmabteilung* (brown
shirts), three major organizations decided to strip the eponym.[18] They prefer
the term "granulomatosis with polyangiitis" to "Wegener's granulomatosis."
Although he never conducted Nazi experiments on humans, 21st-century doctors have determined that Wegener's character and politics make him unde-
serving of an honor for his medical work. Julius Hallervorden, on the other
hand, did do research on the brains of civilians murdered by the Nazis. Thus,
the handy term "Hallervorden-Spatz disease" has been discouraged and "pan-
tothenate kinase-associated neurodegeneration" preferred.

Debate about eponyms is not limited to arguments on priority and appropriateness. Many argue that eponyms, in general, are undesirable. They
point out that confusion can result when multiple disorders are named for
one person like Charcot, Duchenne, or Ramsay Hunt. Another argument
against eponyms stems from the randomness of discovery. So often, two
investigators make similar observations or analyses at about the same time.
As shown earlier, priority is often debatable. In fact, Stigler has proposed
Stigler's Law of Eponymy: "No scientific discovery is named after its original discoverer."[19]

On the other hand, eponyms are good. We are fortunate that "Korsakoff
psychosis" has replaced the Russian's own term, "cerebropathia psychica tox-
aemica," which is polysyllabic and incorrect. Even a long eponym can be better

than the endless arguments about the anatomic or pathologic correctness of competing terms. The artery of Adamkiewicz has become a good term for his "arteria magna spinalis." The eponym avoids arguments about whether the artery should be named for the neighboring vertebra, nerve root, or spinal cord segment, or a combination of them. In sum, "There is no better way to say Foster Kennedy syndrome than simply say Foster Kennedy Syndrome."[20]

Gowers was one who strongly opposed eponyms:[17]

> The direct pyramidal tract is also called the column of Türck; the postero-median column is called the column of Goll, and the postero-external column is called the column of Burdach. I have avoided the use of these terms. This system of nomenclature is full of inconvenience, increasing the difficulties of the student, and leading to frequent mistakes in scientific writings. There are very few observations in medicine regarding which it is not obvious that they would speedily have been made by some other than the actual observer; that it was very much of an accident that they were made by certain individuals. Scientific nomenclature should be itself scientific, not founded upon accidents. However anxious we may be to honour individuals, we have no right to do so at the expense of the convenience of all future generations of learners.

Ironically, Gowers himself is remembered by an eponym. Nicholas J. M. Arts cogently comments:

> Should one follow Gowers' advice then and change this eponym for a descriptive term, for instance, "leg-climbing sign"? Little would be gained. Leg-climbing sign would be a cryptic as Gowers' sign and have lost the implicit remembrance of one of the greatest clinicians in neurological history.[17]

IMAGING AND TERMINOLOGY

Imaging has also led to the popularization of terms little known or unknown before computed tomography (CT) scanning. "Leukoaraiosis" is a term developed as a shorthand for radiolucencies in the white matter near the lateral ventricles. For these same areas, which show as increased signal on magnetic resonance imaging (MRI) scans, the term "chronic white matter changes" is often used. This term is quite nonspecific, and the changes encompassed range from multifocal to bilaterally symmetric. Basically, the radiologist wants a shorthand to say that he sees such changes frequently and that he does not suspect active or serious disease.

Modern imaging has led to new terminology by bringing insight into diseases. The well-demonstrated brain pathology in patients dying from hypertensive encephalopathy had been multiple small-vessel distribution infarcts. With CT scanning and especially with MRI scanning, it became evident that areas of white matter edema could also occur with malignant hypertension and that they would improve after lowering of the blood pressure. These scan findings were often but not always in the parieto-occipital areas. The prevailing term for them is "posterior reversible encephalopathy syndrome" (PRES). I find this term unappealing because the edema is often not posterior, is not always reversible (small areas of infarction can persist), is not always symptomatic, and is not a syndrome. Although every word in the term is incorrect, the acronym often impresses residents that they have found the "answer" to their patient's problem in the radiologist's report.

UNIFORMITY

At a certain point in a career, scientists may take to organizing and joining commissions and committees to come to consensus about various topics. Such group endeavors can make good recommendations. The Birmingham Revision of Basle Nomina Anat recommends that the second cervical vertebra be termed "axis" rather than the competing term "epistropheus." However, such committees can intrude where there is no need. The Federative Committee on Anatomical Terminology states that the preferred term for the peroneal nerve is the fibular nerve. According to Robinson, the committee preferred this term over "peroneal nerve" due to concern that "peroneal" could be confused with the "perineal nerve"! [21] (Note that "peroneal" is basically a Greek-derived word for the Latin derived "fibular.") Is it really that difficult for people with doctoral degrees to distinguish the term describing the perineum from the word "peroneal"?

FINAL COMMENTS

1. If a term is useful it will be used. "Metabolic encephalopathy," for example, is a widely used term in contemporary neurology. It appears to have emerged with no fanfare in the monograph *Diagnosis of Stupor and Coma*. Fred Plum developed a classification of causes of coma, supratentorial, infratentorial, and metabolic. His metabolic encephalopathies comprised hyponatremia, hypercalcemia, and other chemical derangements affecting brain metabolism. Plum was not the first to categorize metabolic disease of the nervous system as a

cause of coma. However, it seems that the specific label "metabolic encephalopathy" was his. Experts are not aware of any prior use of the term (Jerome Posner, MD, and Eelco Wijdicks, MD, in emails, 2016).

2. Successful terms like "aphasia" tend to be shorter. Longer words like "amorphosynthesis," no matter how appropriate, are less likely to catch on. Long terms that can be abbreviated as acronyms can succeed. "ADEM" makes "acute disseminated encephalomyelitis" more likely to remain in the neurologist's vocabulary.

3. A poetic quality can make a term appealing. "Watershed" infarction continues to be used, although "border zone" is a better description of the process. "Oligoclonal" scans nicely, but there is no evidence that several bands on an electrophoresis of cerebrospinal fluid are produced from several clones of cells.

4. Renaming often follows development of new knowledge When one renames a disease or phenomenon, he may thereby become an authority. If current trends continue, however, he is unlikely to have the honor of an eponym.

REFERENCES

1. Campbell FR. *The language of medicine: a manual giving the origin, etymology, pronunciation, and meaning of the technical terms found in medical literature.* New York: Appleton; 1888.

2. Feindel W, ed. The origin and significance of cerebri anatome. In: Willis T. *The anatomy of the brain and nerves.* Birmingham, AL: Gryphon Editions; 1983; 1–53. The Classics of Neurology and Neurosurgery.

3. Bladin CF, Chambers BR, Donnan GA. Confusing stroke terminology: watershed or borderzone infarction? *Stroke.* 1993;24(3):477–478.

4. Landau WM, Nelson DA. Clinical neuromythology XV. Feinting science: Neurocardiogenic syncope and collateral vasovagal confusion. *Neurology.* 1996;46(3):609–618.

5. Osler W. The Gulstonian lectures on malignant endocarditis. *BMJ.* 1885;1(1262):467–470.

6. Rowland LP. Myoglobinuria, 1984. *Can J Neurol Sci.* 1984;11(1):1–13.

7. Campbell WW. *Clinical signs in neurology: a compendium.* Philadelphia, PA: Wolters Kluwer; 2016.

8. Lungu C, Hirtz D, Damiano D, Gross P, Mink JW. Report of a workshop on research gaps in the treatment of cerebral palsy. *Neurology.* 2016;87(12):1293–1298.

9. Landau ME, Campbell WW. Clinical features and electrodiagnosis of ulnar neuropathies. *Phys Med Rehabil Clin N Am.* 2013;24(1):49–66.

10. Layton KF, Kallmes DF, Cloft HJ, Lindell EP, Cox VS. Bovine aortic arch variant in humans: clarification of a common misnomer. *AJNR Am J Neuroradiol.* 2006;27(7):1541–1542.

11. Judson HF. *The eighth day of creation: makers of the revolution in biology.* Plainview, NY: Cold Spring Harbor Press; 1996;605–608.

12. Russell JA, Williams MA, Drogan O. Sedation for the imminently dying: survey results from the AAN Ethics Section. *Neurology.* 2010;74(16):1303–1309.

13. Rady MY, Verheijde JL. Sedation for the imminently dying: survey results from the AAN Ethics Section. *Neurology.* 2010;75(19):1753; author reply 1753–1754.

14. Wall M, Corbett JJ. Revised diagnostic criteria for the pseudotumor cerebri syndrome in adults and children. *Neurology.* 2014;83(2):198–199.

15. Kanner AM, Meador KJ. Remember . . . there is more to epilepsy than seizures! *Neurology.* 2015;85(13):1094–1095.

16. Wijdicks EF. Being comatose: why definition matters. *Lancet Neurol.* 2012;11(8):657–658.

17. Koehler PJ, Bruyn GW, Pearce J. *Neurological eponyms.* New York: Oxford University Press; 2000.

18. Falk RJ, Gross WL, Guillevin L, Hoffman GS, Jayne DR, Jennette JC, Kallenberg CG, et al. Granulomatosis with polyangiitis (Wegener's): an alternative name for Wegener's granulomatosis. *Arthritis Rheum.* 2011;63(4):863–864.

19. Stigler SM. A law of eponymy. In: Gieryn TF, Merton RK, eds. *Science and social structure: a festschift for Robert K. Merton.* New York: New York Academy of Sciences; 1980.

20. Campbell WW. *DeJong's the neurologic examination.* Philadelphia, PA: Wolters Kluwer/Lippincott Williams & Wilkins; 2013.

21. Robinson LR. What do we call that structure? *Muscle Nerve.* 2010;42(6):981; author reply 981.

10

Classifications

"Eventually every system of classification breaks down." This was the teaching of Maurice Victor. The basic problem is that many natural phenomena fail to fit into neat categories. In fact, some diseases defy classification. Syringomyelia, for example, is an enigma to neuropathologists because it does not fit into any standard disease category.

Superimposed on the problem of nature's complexity is the problem of the experts. Doctors disagree about classification. "Taxonomy is described sometimes as a science and sometimes as an art, but really it's a battleground."[1]

Difficulties notwithstanding, we must classify. We classify to aid research, education, and clinical thinking. We classify anatomic structures, and we classify diseases.

NEUROANATOMY

Neuroanatomic classification begins with two categories of nerves: the cranial nerves which exit through apertures in the cranium and the spinal nerves which exit from the spinal column. Generations of medical students have found this distinction useful. However, this classification is not based on a fundamental biologic distinction. The spinal cord and the brainstem are a continuous structure. Cranial nerve 11 comes off the spinal cord, courses into the cranium, and exits the skull through the jugular foramen. The second cranial nerve is not a nerve at all. It is an elongated tract of the central nervous system (CNS).

Our current classification of 12 pairs of cranial nerves was not self-evident. Galen recognized seven pairs of cranial nerves, the first being our optic nerves. He did not recognize cranial nerves 4 and 6. He considered the fifth sensory and motor roots as separate nerves. He considered our cranial nerves 7 and 8, which together traverse the internal auditory canal, to be one nerve. Likewise, our nerves 9, 10, and 11, all coursing through the jugular foramen, he classified as one nerve (one foramen, one nerve). Benedetti (1445–1525) was the first to label the olfactory tract as a cranial nerve. (Galen had considered it a part of the brain, not a nerve.) Willis also accepted the olfactory tract as cranial nerve I.[2] His classification of nine cranial nerves begins to resemble our own except that he, as Galen, continued to group our nerves 7 and 8 as one nerve and our nerves 9, 10, and 11 as one.

Finally Sömmering (1755–1830) proposed the classification of 12 cranial nerves that we use today.[2] Our classification is not perfect, and one could argue for numerous changes. What are often referred to as cranial nerves 1 and 2 are not nerves at all; they are elongated parts of the brain. The accessory nerve is not cranial in origin. The nervus intermedius, which leaves the brainstem separately from cranial nerve 7 and is considered part of it, could be viewed as a separate nerve. Left out of our classification is the nervus terminalis. It has been largely ignored by clinicians due to its small size and lack of easily testable function. One might call this nerve 0, but there is no zero in the Roman numeral system that is used for cranial nerves. Hence came the suggestion that it be called nerve N (for the Latin nulla).[3] Including nerve N and the nervus intermedius and subdividing the trigeminal nerve into its roots would have given us 16 cranial nerves instead of 12.[2]

Nevertheless, it is sensible to continue the current classification of cranial nerves. All are long, narrow protrusions from the brain or upper spinal cord. All are bilateral structures as they exit the skull or extend toward the foramina that allow connection to extracranial structures. While it is true that some are tracts, not nerves, some originate from the spinal cord rather than the brainstem, and some emerge as multiple rootlets, the current system has proved its utility for clinical work over the course of centuries.

DISEASES

Writing down a classification of a family of diseases helps one to think about the subject. As new information emerges, one can reassess what he has written. A good example of this process is the evolving classification of the demyelinative diseases in Adams and Victor's *Principles of Neurology*.[4] In the first edition (1977), one finds:

  I. Multiple sclerosis
    A. Chronic relapsing encephalomyelopathic form
    B. Acute multiple sclerosis
    C. Neuromyelitis optica

II. Acute disseminated encephalomyelitis
    A. Following viral infection
    B. Postvaccinial

III. Schilder's diffuse cerebral sclerosis and concentric sclerosis of Balo
IV. Acute and subacute necrotizing hemorrhagic leukoencephalitis
    A. Acute encephalopathic form (Hurst)
    B. Subacute myelopathy?
    C. Acute brain purpura (acute pericapillary encephalorrhagia)?

By the sixth edition (1997), the classification had evolved. Subacute necrotizing myelopathy was no longer questionable. Another questioned entity, acute brain purpura, no longer appears as a demyelinative disease. It is discussed elsewhere in the book.

By the seventh edition, there had been further change:

I. Multiple sclerosis
    A. Chronic relapsing encephalomyelopathic form
    B. Acute multiple sclerosis
    C. Schilder's diffuse cerebral sclerosis and diffuse concentric
       sclerosis of Balo

II. Neuromyelitis optica
III. Acute disseminated encephalomyelitis
    A. Following infections by virus, mycoplasma, or rickettsia
    B. Post-vaccinial

IV. Acute and subacute necrotizing hemorrhagic encephalitis
    A. Acute encephalopathic form (Hurst)
    B. Subacute necrotizing myelopathy

In this later classification, neuromyelitis optica is no longer a subheading of multiple sclerosis; it has its own Roman numeral as a major category. Schilder's disease no longer merits its own Roman numeral and is viewed as a subset of multiple sclerosis. Acute disseminated encephalomyelitis is now recognized to follow infections other than viral ones.

These sequential editions show classification to be an ongoing process. I make no attempt here to discuss whether the later classifications are better than the earlier ones. What we are seeing is the continuing process of trying to make sense of the disorders, to determine if and how they are related.

Whether diseases should be classified by "lumping" (fewer categories) or "split-ting" (numerous categories) remains problematic in the era of molecular biol-ogy. Disorders of mitochondrial DNA (mtDNA), if lumped, make a "swamp of heterogeneous multisystemic disorders."[5] The splitters define several well-defined syndromes such as Kearns-Sayre syndrome (KSS), chronic progressive external ophthalmoplegia (CPEO) and mitochondrial encephalopathy, lactic acidosis and stroke-like episodes (MELAS). Some of these acronymic diseases are due to large-scale deletions, some to transfer RNA mutations, and some to mutations in protein-coding genes. Some of these mtDNA disease phenotypes can be asso-ciated with multiple different mtDNA mutations. Furthermore, some patients' phenotypes are combinations of two standard acronymic syndromes. Whether the doctor is a lumper or splitter, there will be problems with classification.

Similarly problematic is the classification of degenerative brain diseases. On the one hand, there are doctors who seek a common denominator for them all. On the other hand, there are doctors who classify brain degenerations in many categories, subcategories. and overlap syndromes.

One current attempt at simplification comes from the concept of "tauopa-thy." Tau protein accumulates in the brain in an insoluble hyperphosphory-lated form. Sharing this pathologic feature are progressive supranuclear palsy, frontotemporal dementia, corticobasal degeneration, and progressive nonflu-ent aphasia. Although the standard "splitter's" view is that these are separate diseases, the "lumpers" consider these diseases part of a clinical spectrum of conditions with a common pathologic denominator.[6]

In Parkinson disease, many attempts have been made at classifying sub-groups. For example, a subtype "may be based on motor features (tremor dom-inant), cognitive features, age at onset, rate of progression or a combination of these."[7] To a large extent, these subtypes are based on clinical features, not biomarkers or pathology. Aside from descriptive value, the benefit of such a classification has yet to be shown by differences in response to therapy or some other biological variable.

Primary progressive aphasia, described by Pick but today less often known by its eponym, is a heterogeneous group of aphasias. Associated is frontotem-poral atrophy. A suggested classification into three subgroups—semantic, agrammatic/nonfluent, and logopenic—has not worked well. Some cases do not fit clearly in any clinical category. These proposed clinical groups "do not correspond to specific histopathologies. The relationships among phe-notypes, genotypes, anatomic locations, and neuropathology eludes a simple organization."[8]

In kind, Maurice Victor taught that "the more that one probes at the indi-vidual attributes" of a disease, the more the classification breaks down. "Finite subdivisions are not justified" (Maurice Victor, MD, in conversation, c. 1976). In classification, we must strike a balance between detail and clinical utility. A clinician may prefer a classification of stroke into large-vessel atherosclerosis, small-vessel occlusive disease, cardiac source, and other causes.[9] The simplicity of this classification is its advantage. The problem with this classification is that it masks complexity; "other" causes of stroke include unusual large-vessel diseases, uncommon small-vessel diseases, and various systemic diseases.

OVERALL CLASSIFICATION
OF NEUROLOGICAL DISEASES

The International Classification of Disease (ICD) was developed for tracking morbidity and mortality statistics in different countries. This World Health Organization document is used for epidemiology in almost every country.

The United States is exceptional in adopting this public health classification for charge coding, a use for which it was never intended. Successive editions of the ICD have become so detailed as to be cumbersome for billing documentation. Taking into account the explosion of knowledge of genes and antibodies, newer editions of the ICD may "result in increased granularity. . . . A balance needs to be struck between inclusive totality and clinical utility."[10] In preparation for new editions of the ICD, the neurologists have found that each approach to classification—genetic, anatomical, clinical, or pathological—has proved contentious in committee.

ORGANIZATION OF A TEXTBOOK

The table of contents of a neurology textbook is basically a classification of all neurological knowledge. Gowers's *A Manual of Disease of the Nervous System* was divided into five parts: general symptomatology, diseases of the nerves, diseases of the spinal cord, diseases of the brain, and general and functional diseases. The last part included movement disorders, epilepsy, vertigo, and headache.

Much of what Gowers called functional, Wilson's *Manual of Diseases of the Nervous System* discusses in two main parts. In a section on disease conditions of uncertain nature, there is discussion of epilepsy and migraine. In a section on the neuroses, there is exposition on movement disorders and disorders of micturition and defecation.

In 1977, Adams and Victor published *Principles of Neurology,* with its classification of neurological knowledge:[4]

1. Cardinal manifestations of neurologic disease
2. Major categories of neurologic disease
3. Diseases of muscle
4. Psychiatric disorders

In later editions, they revised their classification: diseases of peripheral nerve and muscle were grouped in one part. Finally, in the fifth edition, they grouped diseases of spinal cord, peripheral nerve, and muscle into one part because the spinal cord, nerves, and muscle are intimately related, especially in electrophysiology. After much thought and many editions, the authors concluded that this was the most effective educational grouping of chapters.

Certainly there is no single way to classify neurological knowledge. More important than organization is the clarity of the exposition. However, excellent organization facilitates clear thinking in the student of neurology.

PSYCHIATRY

The less we know about the cause of disorders, the more difficult it is to classify them meaningfully. Psychiatric disorders are a good example of this problem. By mid-20th century, the *Diagnostic And Statistical Manual*[11] (DSM-I) was published by the American Psychiatric Association. This reference and its successor (DSM-II) were basically "glossaries of psychiatric diagnostic terminology."[12] DSM-III was a new kind of volume, aimed at improving the reliability of psychiatric diagnosis. It specified diagnostic criteria. DSM-5 has changed the classification.[13] For example, hypochondriasis, pain disorder, somatization disorder, and undifferentiated somatoform disorder were condensed into a single category, somatic symptom disorder. Bereavement was reclassified under major depressive disorder. These and other changes have not been based on new data. For more than a half century, some diagnostic categories have been voted out and later back into the DSM. This is not exactly science.

An alternative psychiatric classification has been advanced by McHugh. He suggests classifying psychiatric disorders into four "comprehensible clusters": brain diseases, personality dimensions, motivated behaviors, and life encounters.[14,15] In the first group, he includes people who have a disease or a proposed disease of the brain, such as schizophrenia or bipolar disorder. The second group consists of patients who deviate to an extreme in a human disposition or capacity, such as intellect, emotional stability, and extroversion. The third group consists of "those who adopt a behavior that has become a fixed and warped way of life," such as alcoholism, drug addiction, or anorexia nervosa. The final cluster relates to life encounters like bereavement, home-sickness, or post-traumatic stress disorder.

Such a classification allows the doctor to organize his thinking and research. It does not deny that there may be a biologic predisposition to bereavement (life encounter), alcoholism (motivated behavior), or borderline personality (personality dimension). Nor does it deny that one patient may suffer from more than one of these types of problem.

More difficult than classification in neurology, psychiatric classification suffers from a dearth of pathology to facilitate categorization. Hence, a practical clinical grouping, such as that suggested by McHugh, is the best that can be constructed at present.

CONCLUSION

Hughlings Jackson stated that there are two types of classification, that of the gardener and that of the botanist. The gardener needs something for daily work, an empirical classification. He thinks in terms of "trees, shrubs and flowers" and whether plants are "fit for food, for ornament etc."[16] The botanist is a scientist who classifies existing knowledge in a way that shows fundamental relationships and that facilitates the accommodation of new information. He may think of deciduous plants and conifers as groups, unrelated to whether they are edible or decorative and unrelated to whether or not we consider them trees.

Neurologists are sometimes like the botanist and sometimes like the gardener. We need a way of thinking about extant scientific knowledge. Like the botanist, we must distinguish the focal seizures of a post-traumatic epileptic from the absence attacks of a person with hereditary, generalized spike-wave discharges. On the other hand, like the gardener, we may have to give an anticonvulsant medicine to a patient for seizures whether or not we have determined the physiology or cause in a given case.

To generalize, we can best use our evolving classifications if we remember the words of Gowers: "Nature, indeed, is prone to ignore our divisions, and to blend that which we distinguish." [17]

REFERENCES

1. Bryson B. *A short history of nearly everything.* New York: Broadway Books; 2004.
2. O'Rahilly R. On counting cranial nerves. *Acta Anat (Basel).* 1988;133(1):3–4.
3. Vilensky JA. The neglected cranial nerve: nervus terminalis (cranial nerve N). *Clin Anat.* 2014;27(1):46–53.
4. Adams RD, Victor M. *Principles of neurology.* New York: McGraw Hill; 1977.

5. DiMauro S, Schon EA, Carelli V, Hirano M. The clinical maze of mitochondrial neurology. *Nat Rev Neurol.* 2013;9(8):429–444.
6. Bouchard M, Suchowersky O. Tauopathies: one disease or many? *Can J Neurol Sci.* 2011;38(4):547–556.
7. Marras C, Lang A. Parkinson's disease subtypes: lost in translation? *J Neurol Neurosurg Psychiatry.* 2013;84(4):409–415.
8. Drachman DA. The taxonomy of primary progressive aphasia: it walks and quacks like a duck . . . but which duck? *Neurology.* 2011;76(11):942–943.
9. Amarenco P, Bogousslavsky J, Caplan LR, Donnan GA, Hennerici MG. New approach to stroke subtyping: the A-S-C-O (phenotypic) classification of stroke. *Cerebrovasc Dis.* 2009;27(5):502–508.
10. Shakir R, Rajakulendran S. The 11th revision of the International Classification of Diseases (ICD): the neurological perspective. *JAMA Neurol.* 2013;70(11):1353–1354.
11. American Psychiatric Association. *Diagnostic and statistical manual: mental disorders.* Arlington, VA: American Psychiatric Association Publishing; 1952.
12. McCarron RM. The DSM-5 and the art of medicine: certainly uncertain. *Ann Intern Med.* 2013;159(5):360–361.
13. American Psychiatric Association. *Diagnostic and statistical manual: mental disorders.* 5th ed. Arlington, VA: American Psychiatric Association Publishing; 2013.
14. McHugh PR. Striving for coherence: psychiatry's efforts over classification. *JAMA.* 2005;293(20):2526–2528.
15. McHugh PR, Slavney PR. Mental illness: comprehensive evaluation or checklist? *N Engl J Med.* 2012;366(20):1853–1855.
16. Wolf P. Of cabbages and kings: some considerations on classifications, diagnostic schemes, semiology, and concepts. *Epilepsia.* 2003;44(1):1-4-13.
17. Gowers WR. Alecture on the pains of tabes. *Br Med J.* 1905 Jan 7;(2297):1–5.

11

Causation

What is it that we talk about when we talk about cause? Treponema pallidum can cause tabes dorsalis. Because this disease does not occur with other organisms, the spirochete is considered a necessary cause. The polio virus is well known to cause poliomyelitis, but other viruses can cause the same clinico-pathologic syndrome; that is, poliomyelitis can occur without the polio virus. In other words, the polio virus is a sufficient but not necessary cause of the disease. This distinction between necessary and sufficient causes has long proved useful in discussions of causation.

There are causes of disease that are neither necessary nor sufficient. They contribute to the development of a disease but cannot by themselves cause the disease. Living one's childhood and adolescence in Scotland increases a person's probability of developing multiple sclerosis, but living in this region, far from the equator, is neither necessary nor sufficient to cause the disease. This geographical predisposition is a probabilistic cause which shows its effect in combination with other probabilistic causes, known and unknown.[1]

Some dispute the notion of causes. They propose a concept of "contributory factors,"[2] another way of saying that all causes are probabilistic. This approach may be appropriate for analyzing a very general diagnosis like "perinatal brain damage." When the diagnosis is more specific (e.g., kernicterus), it is more likely that we can identify a truly necessary or sufficient cause.

In the absence of experimental evidence for cause, we rely on observational information. Observational study may be prospective or retrospective (case-control study). The retrospective study compares control patients and patients with a particular disease in an effort to identify an antecedent cause. Such studies rely on records and recall, which is hard to validate. A prospective study, often considered the gold standard, has its own disadvantages. Prospective studies require a much larger patient population, and they take a long time and a lot of money.[3]

For demonstrating causation there stand two landmark standards, that of Henle-Koch and that of Bradford Hill. The Henle-Koch postulates were the early guide for proof of cause in infectious disease.[4,5] Subsequent postulate-based proofs of disease causation have been modeled on Henle-Koch. The Bradford Hill criteria became the guide for determining whether an environmental variable was the cause of a disease.[6] Use of postulates and criteria can strongly support that an association is causal. Failure to fulfill postulates and criteria, however, can never exclude a causal relationship.

HENLE-KOCH POSTULATES

Henle-Koch's postulates state that a suspect organism must be found in all cases of the disease, that it can be isolated and grown in culture, and that inoculation of a pure culture into humans or animals reproduces the disease. No control group is required. Fulfilling these requirements, especially with a control inoculation group, strongly supports causation.

The Henle-Koch postulates were not useful for viral disease. Rivers proposed two conditions to establish a specific relationship of a virus to a disease:[4,5]

1. The virus must be regularly associated with the disease.
2. The virus must be found in the sick person not as an incidental finding.

The latter requirement might be shown by appropriate antibody responses. Others emphasized that development of a successful vaccine provided convincing evidence for a causal relationship. In virology, causation can be considered proved without fulfilling any of Koch's postulates.

The long latencies in slow viral disease required new ideas about proof of causation. Johnson and Gibbs set criteria for causation as:[7]

1. Consistency in transmission of the disease to experimental animals or consistent recovery of the virus in cell cultures
2. Consistent serial transmission or consistent demonstration of the agent in the appropriate brain cells
3. Control studies in tissues of unaffected patients showing that the virus is not ubiquitous

Modern technology allows DNA sequence recognition by polymerase chain reaction to identify the presence of an organism in diseased tissue.[8] A convincing relationship of the organism to disease is shown when the sequence is present in extraordinary quantity or when the sequence is present in a series of patients with the disease and absent in patients without the disease. The causation role of the Whipple disease bacillus was supported by this type of evidence. Henle-Koch postulates 2 and 3 were never met for Whipple disease.

Spongiform encephalopathies like scrapie and Creutzfeldt-Jakob disease are transmissible. Prusiner has advanced considerable evidence that the diseases can be transmitted without nucleic acids.[9] He has demonstrated that the material which transmits the disease has biochemical and physical properties of protein and has hence named the disease-carrying material proteinaceous infectious agents ("prions"). Richard Johnson stated that proof of the prion concept has one critical step: extraction of a purified protein to show "that it and it alone is infectious."[10] One might call this Johnson's postulate. Walker et al. have gone further in delineating postulates for establishing an infectious protein as the cause of a disease:[11]

1. The protein must be invariably present in a disease-specific form and arrangement in the diseased tissue.
2. The physicochemical characteristics that confer infectivity on a specific protein must be established.
3. The characteristics that render the host susceptible to infection by a specific proteinaceous agent must be established.
4. The disease process must be induced in a susceptible organism by the pure agent in its infectious form.
5. The protein must be recovered in its infectious form from the animal that was experimentally infected with the pure agent.

The Henle-Koch approach has been applied outside the realm of infectious disease. Witebsky suggested postulates on this model for proving a disease to be autoimmune.[12] Thinking only of antibody-mediated disease, he listed criteria to be fulfilled to demonstrate autoimmune causation:

1. Demonstration of antibody in the human
2. Recognition of the specific antigen against which the antibody is directed
3. Production of antibodies against the same antigen in experimental animals
4. Reproduction of the pathology of the human disease in an actively sensitized experimental animals

Later, this approach to autoimmune disease was modified to accommodate knowledge of cellular immunity.[13]

Gershon similarly developed postulates to challenge himself in studying serotonin as a possible neurotransmitter in the enteric nervous system.[14] If serotonin were a neurotransmitter, he postulated that it should:

1. Be present in the nerve endings at the proposed sites of neurotransmission
2. Mimic the effects of the natural neurotransmitter
3. Actually be released when the nerves that contain it are stimulated
4. Be rendered ineffective by blocking the action of serotonin or depleting it

Gershon was able to establish the role of serotonin neurotransmission in the enteric nervous system by experiments that met these postulates.[14] His work is an example of a Henle-Koch approach being useful outside the fields of infection, pathology, and immunology.

BRADFORD HILL CRITERIA

Publication of the Bradford Hill criteria was another landmark in thinking on medical causation. His interest was the field of environmental and occupational medicine. Bradford Hill pointed out aspects of an association that one should "consider before deciding that the most likely interpretation of it is causation."[6] In other words, he proposed guidelines for thinking through a problem before rendering a judgment. He offered no strict rules for excluding or proving causation in a given situation.

Bradford Hill suggests analyzing nine aspects of an association:

1. Strength of association
2. Consistency of the association in different studies and places
3. Specificity of an association
4. Temporal relationship of the disease and the putative cause
5. A clear dose–response curve (In other words, a biological gradient favors a causal relationship.)
6. Biological plausibility
7. Coherence with our knowledge of the disease
8. Experimental confirmation (the strongest support for a causation hypothesis)
9. Analogy to known phenomena

In neurology, the Bradford Hill criteria are particularly helpful in studying toxic neuropathies and encephalopathies.[15] However, the criteria have influenced thinking on causation of other types of disease.

STATISTICAL SIGNIFICANCE AND CAUSATION

Tests of significance are useful guides to remind doctors that chance can affect the outcome of a study that compares two or more groups. It is a mistake to ignore study results simply because statistical significance has not been shown. Without any statistical method, one can draw meaningful conclusions when the differences between groups are very obvious. In addition, the presence of statistical significance is irrelevant if the difference between two groups is "too small to be of practical importance."[6] In other words "statistical significance is neither necessary nor sufficient for substantive significance."[16] Statistical significance should not be a straight-jacket for a neurologist tryng to determine causation. A small case series is sometimes more revealing than a large, prospective, controlled study.

Kenneth Rothman proselytized for limiting the role of statistical significance in thinking about causation. Having had limited success, he finally started his own journal and set his own editorial policy:

> When writing for *Epidemiology*, you can . . . enhance your prospects if you omit tests of statistical significance . . .. In *Epidemiology*, we do not publish them at all . . .. We discourage the use of this type of thinking in the data analysis, such as in the use of stepwise regression. We also would like to see the interpretation of a study based not on statistical significance, or lack of it, for one or more study variables, but rather on careful quantitative consideration of the data in light of competing explanations for the findings. For example, we prefer a researcher to consider whether the magnitude of an estimated effect could be readily explained by uncontrolled confounding or selection biases, rather than simply to offer the uninspired interpretation that the estimated effect is "significant."[17]

CAUSATION IN COURT

In torts, there are three steps in determining whether an exposure caused a neurologic problem.[18] One must determine whether the plaintiff has a disorder, whether the agent under discussion has been proved to be able to cause the disease in question, and whether the exposure did, in fact, cause the neurologic problem in that particular plaintiff.

Diagnosing whether a person has a disease is standard activity for a neurologist. If a patient has parkinsonism or a biopsy-proven meningioma, the diagnosis is straightforward in the clinic or in the legal arena. However, when a psychologist alleges the presence of encephalopathy from a battery of psychological tests, there is a challenge to the neurologist. There are many subtests to psychological tests. When a person tests below average on some subtests and above average on others, a psychologist may state that the low scores on scattered subtests indicate brain damage. A neurologist may have to judge whether the psychologist's diagnosis of encephalopathy is appropriate. One might doubt the psychologist's opinion, for example, when the "brain-damaged" plaintiff is both an honor student and a varsity athlete.

When the diagnosis of a disorder is clear, one must determine whether exposure to a physical or chemical agent has been proved to be able to cause that disorder. A migraineur may believe that years of drinking soft drinks with artificial sweeteners caused his episodic headaches. A multiple sclerosis patient may attribute his disease to a fall on an icy sidewalk. In such cases, the lack of good scientific or medical literature showing that the proposed cause can actually produce the neurologic problem in question is as great a weakness in court as it is in the clinic.

The third step in thinking about medicolegal causation is to analyze whether an exposure in a particular plaintiff did cause that person's neurologic condition. For example, a diabetic with peripheral neuropathy may work at a business where an organic solvent is used in manufacturing. She works in an office area. She may believe that the solvent has caused her neuropathy. However, her medical records show evidence of diabetic polyneuropathy prior to her taking a job at this factory. In addition, her exposure to solvents is minimal in the office area where she sits. Furthermore, no other worker in the office or the factory areas has developed neuropathy. Although the solvent used can cause polyneuropathy, the neurologist would likely judge it more likely than not that the neuropathy of this particular patient was unrelated to the solvent.

The neurological thought process is similar in the court room and the clinic. We always rely on evidence and judgment. What differs is the standard of evidence. In civil law, a "more likely than not" determination is adequate to establish causation. In medicine, we expect evidence that allows us to make a stronger statement about causation.

CONCLUSION

What we consider good evidence for establishing causation will change as our technology advances. New postulates and criteria will emerge. Rivers taught that making good judgments about the evidence requires, in addition to clear thinking, the priceless attribute of common sense.[5] As new diseases are recognized, the neurologist must require that sufficient evidence be accumulated "to make a case beyond reasonable doubt for a cause and effect relationship."[7]

REFERENCES

1. Parascandola M, Weed DL. Causation in epidemiology. *J Epidemiol Community Health.* 2001;55(12):905–912.
2. Dammann O, Leviton A. The challenge of causal inference. *Ann Neurol.* 2010;68(5):770.
3. Schlesselman JJ, Stolley PD. *Case-control studies: design, conduct, analysis.* New York: Oxford University Press; 1982.
4. Evans AS. *Causation and disease: a chronological journey.* New York: Plenum Medical Book Company; 1993.
5. Evans AS. Causation and disease: the Henle-Koch postulates revisited. *Yale J Biol Med.* 1976;49(2):175–195.
6. Hill AB. The environment and disease: association or causation? *Proc R Soc Med.* 1965;58:295–300.
7. Johnson RT, Gibbs CJ. Editorial: Koch's postulates and slow infections of the nervous system. *Arch Neurol.* 1974;30(1):36–38.
8. Fredricks DN, Relman DA. Sequence-based identification of microbial pathogens: a reconsideration of Koch's postulates. *Clin Microbiol Rev.* 1996;9(1):18–33.
9. Pruisiner SB. *Madness and memory: the discovery of prions: A new biological principle of disease.* New Haven, CT: Yale University Press; 2014.
10. Johnson RT. The novel nature of scrapie. *Trends Neurosci.* 1982;5:413–415.
11. Walker L, Levine H, Jucker M. Koch's postulates and infectious proteins. *Acta Neuropathol.* 2006;112(1):1–4.
12. Witebsky E, Rose NR, Terplan K, Paine JR, Egan RW. Chronic thyroiditis and autoimmunization. *J Am Med Assoc.* 1957;164(13):1439–1447.
13. Rose NR, Bona C. Defining criteria for autoimmune diseases (Witebsky's postulates revisited). *Immunol Today.* 1993;14(9):426–430.
14. Gershon M. *The second brain: a groundbreaking new understanding of nervous disorders of the stomach and intestine.* New York: HarperCollins; 2003.
15. Morrison B, Chaudhry V. Medication, toxic, and vitamin-related neuropathies. *Continuum (Minneap Minn).* 2012;18(1):139–160.
16. Ziliak ST, McClosky DN. *The cult of statistical significance: how the standard error costs us jobs, justice, and lives.* Ann Arbor: University of Michigan Press; 2008.
17. Rothman KJ. Writing for epidemiology. *Epidemiology.* 1998;9(3):333–337.
18. Gots RE. Medical causation and expert testimony. *Regul Toxicol Pharmacol.* 1986;6(2):95–102.

12

Asymmetry

Neurologists encounter asymmetry daily. They regularly see asymmetry of the pupil diameter. Alpha rhythm amplitude differences are frequently found between the right and left sides on a scalp recording. Within limited ranges, these asymmetries are "physiologic." Comparing compound muscle action potentials on the left and the right, one expects asymmetry. One never considers a response abnormally low on one side unless it is less than 50% of that obtained by stimulation of the contralateral nerve. This chapter comprises discussion of several topics about central nervous system asymmetries and their importance to the neurologist.

ANATOMIC AND FUNCTIONAL ASYMMETRY

Brains are not perfectly symmetric. Whether one examines external morphology, white matter tracts, arterial supply, venous drainage, or the ventricular system, one may find asymmetry in a given brain. Not all of the asymmetries are important. However, neurologists must be aware of the anatomic asymmetries that occur.

Normal faces are symmetric in the sense that there are two eyes, two ears, one midline nose, and one midline mouth. On a given face, however, the nasolabial folds, palpebral fissures, and other features may be asymmetric. The normal brain is symmetric in the same way that faces are: there are two frontal lobes, two sylvian fissures, two calcarine fissures, and one corpus callosum. The two hemispheres are similar in weight and volume. Nevertheless, any given brain will show asymmetries. Sometimes the right hemisphere protrudes anteriorly beyond the left, and the left hemisphere extends more posteriorly than the right. (These asymmetries and the associated asymmetries, of the skull, are termed *petalia*.) As a result of these asymmetries, the anterior portion of the right hemisphere may twist toward the left and the posterior portion of the left hemisphere may twist toward the right.[1] This "Yakovlevian torque" can be observed on axial brain images. This pattern of asymmetry can be detected in the fetus as well as the adult.[2] There is some evidence that patients with situs inversus totalis of the viscera also have reversal of the standard hemispheric asymmetry.[3]

Asymmetry of the cerebral ventricles can be developmental and of no importance. For example, the ependyma overlying the head of the caudate nucleus and the ependyma under the corpus callosum can stick to each other during development. Although the resulting coaptation, if asymmetric, can be eye-catching, it is asymptomatic. Coaptation can also occur in the temporal horn. Even without coaptation, there can be mild differences in the size of the right and left lateral ventricles. Most conspicuous and common is asymmetry of the occipital horns. The occipital horns are the last portions of the ventricles to appear in both the evolution of mammals and in the development of the human embryo. Thus, it is not surprising that the occipital horn can be normally absent on one side or the other.[4,5] Ultrasonography reveals occipital horn asymmetry in utero[6] and in the neonate.[7] Such florid asymmetry is of no importance.

The surface structure of the hemispheres also reveals asymmetries. Asymmetry of the planum temporale has generated the greatest interest. In each half of the cerebrum, a cut in the plane of the Sylvian fissure allows inspection of the upper surface of the temporal lobe. In 65% of brains it is larger on the left than on the right. It is larger on the right in 11% of cases.[8] Wada's study of 100 adult and 100 fetal brains confirmed that the left temporal planum is, more often than not, larger than the right.[9] He also found asymmetry in the posterior regions of the Sylvian fissures. In a study of 36 brains of right-handed adults, the right fissure angulated sharply up into the parietal area in 25. On the left, the fissure continued back without this upward bend. The lack of up-angulation on the left is associated with the larger planum temporale on that side; the upward bend of the fissure on the right is linked with a larger inferior parietal area.[10] Planum temporale asymmetry has also been described in the chimpanzee.[11] Sylvian fissure asymmetry has been found in monkeys.[12]

These anatomical studies have been motivated largely by interest in the functional asymmetry of the cerebral hemispheres. It was wondered whether hemispheric dominance for handedness or language could have a gross anatomical basis. It turns out that these asymmetries are unrelated to handedness.[13] Almost all patients have left hemisphere language dominance. However, only 65% of patients have a larger planum on the left.

Not only does functional asymmetry correlate poorly with anatomic asymmetry, but also functional asymmetries do not correlate with each other.[14]

The typical person has language and handedness dominance in the left hemisphere. However, 10% of right-handed aphasics have a lesion in the right hemisphere, and 30% of sinistral aphasics have a lesion in the left hemisphere. Likewise, ocular dominance (sighting a gun) bears no simple relationship to handedness.[15]

There remains the question as to why there is functional asymmetry superimposed on relatively symmetric brain morphology. Why does a person usually have language function concentrated in one cerebral hemisphere or another? Kinsbourne states that neurologic symmetry is most useful for the movement of somatic muscles that need to respond to sensory stimuli from both the right and the left. Asymmetry for manual dexterity became superimposed. "Whereas language originated in a motor context, it is not in itself deployed toward specific points in ambient space."[16] Kinsbourne continues:

> If we accept that it is bisymmetry which develops in response to an adaptive imperative, we can easily explain why language does not conform to that same pattern. Its organization was not influenced in this way; there was no specific need for bisymmetry, and so no need for bisymmetrical language representation to evolve. Therefore like any other structure not forced into the bisymmetrical mode, language-related cerebral cortex conformed to the less constrained asymmetrical state, which in humans happens to be left sided in a species-specific manner.[16]

At the microscopic level, asymmetries can be found between the left and right hemispheres in the motor cortex, visual cortex, Wernicke area, and Broca area.[17] There can be asymmetry of the fraction of tissue occupied by neuronal branches and cell bodies. There can be asymmetry of neuronal cell number or complexity of dendritic branches. This population-level asymmetry may be meaningful, but it bears no demonstrable relationship to functional asymmetry. There is variation in such asymmetries from one individual to another. In sum, there is no simple relationship of brain asymmetry and functional asymmetry. "Those who seek for anatomical correlates of unilateral hemisphere dominance may be up against the possibility that the anatomy of the hemispheres is entirely irrelevant to this problem."[18]

The extreme form of gross morphologic asymmetry is the patient with only one hemisphere. Despite the absence of the entire right diencephalon and telencephalon and right microphthalmia, near normal vision was present in both hemifields.[19] In other words, the left eye's nasal retinal fibers and its temporal retinal fibers projected to the ipsilateral lateral geniculate and visual cortex. This case indicates that gross asymmetry of the hemispheres does not imply gross functional loss. Developmental rerouting of what would have been chiasmal fibers and adaptation of higher visual centers to the atypical retinal projection allowed vision in both hemifields of the good eye!

Asymmetry in the cerebral white matter has been revealed by anatomical methods and magnetic resonance methods. These investigations have focused on large white matter tracts, the arcuate fasciculus and the optic radiation. Meyer's loop is the portion of the optic radiation that passes forward into the temporal lobe before heading back toward the occipital pole. Investigators randomly selected 60 epileptic patients whose anterior temporal lobes had been resected. Pre- and postoperative visual fields and brain magnetic resonance imaging (MRI) scans were studied. Unrelated to the size of the resection, visual field defects were found 3.5 times more frequently with left-side resection than with surgery on the right. This result suggests that, in most patients, Meyer's loop extends more anteriorly in the left hemisphere than it does in the right.[20] It is not only the geniculo-calcarine tract that shows asymmetry. MRI tractography showed that the volume of the arcuate fasciculus was greater on the left than the right in 80% of right-handed people.[21]

The spinal cord is asymmetric in nearly 75% of cases. Of these asymmetric cords, the right side is larger in three-quarters. The asymmetry is due to the crossed lateral corticospinal tract and the uncrossed anterior corticospinal tract, which both contain more fibers on the larger side of the cord. [22]

DISEASE

Asymptomatic developmental asymmetries can become important when disease is superimposed on congenital vascular variants. The vertebral artery, for example, is often hypoplastic on one side. Occlusion of the hypoplastic vessel will likely not cause a stroke. In these cases, the dominant vertebral provides most of the blood flow to the basilar artery. If, however, the dominant vertebral artery becomes occluded, severe ischemia can result in the distribution of the posterior circulation. Had the vertebral arteries been symmetric, no stroke may have occurred. In the venous circulation, there is an analogous situation. The transverse sinus is typically much larger on one side. Thrombosis of this dominant channel can easily spread back into the sagittal sinus and cause a severe neurological deficit. In less severe cases, thrombosis of the dominant transverse sinus can cause headache and increased intracranial pressure. Occlusion of the smaller transverse sinus might cause no symptoms. Had the transverse sinuses been of equal bore and flow, the thrombosis of one may have been less symptomatic than the occlusion of a dominant sinus.

In generalized disorders like idiopathic increased intracranial pressure, we would expect to have symmetric neurologic effects. Underlying anatomic asymmetries, however, may result in asymmetric manifestations. Truly unilateral papilledema is the best example.[23] Very asymmetric papilledema also occurs.[24] This clinical asymmetry has been attributed to underlying asymmetry of the optic nerve sheath.[25] The side with the larger optic nerve sheath develops optic disc edema earlier and more markedly than its counterpart.[24] With the advent of the coronal MRI scans of the orbits, it has become evident that normal optic nerves often have asymmetric sheaths. Thus, the hypothesis of Hayreh is plausible. Other anatomic asymmetries presumably underlie the occurrence of unilateral sixth-nerve palsy or other one-sided manifestations of increased intracranial pressure, such as unilateral seventh-nerve paresis or unilateral tinnitus.

There remain many opportunities for an investigator. For example, a genetic basis for brain asymmetry should be sought. The study of twins by Bartley and Weinberger[26] shows that in vivo investigation of brain variability is feasible, as has the investigation of Thompson et al.[27] With cross-sectional brain imaging, multiple generations in a family could be easily analyzed for hereditary asymmetry.

Over the decades, awareness of cerebral asymmetries has been important for the neurologist. In the era of the pneumoencephalogram, it was important to recognize a ventricular asymmetry as being due to coaptation rather than mass effect. When auditory evoked potentials were in vogue, it was essential to know that an asymmetric result could be caused by a normal asymmetry in temporoparietal anatomy rather than a disease process. The neurologist will always need to be alert to the presence of normal asymmetries in the central and peripheral nervous system.

REFERENCES

1. Toga AW, Thompson PM. Mapping brain asymmetry. *Nat Rev Neurosci.* 2003;4(1):37–48.
2. Weinberger DR, Luchins DJ, Morihisa J, Wyatt RJ. Asymmetrical volumes of the right and left frontal and occipital regions of the human brain. *Ann Neurol.* 1982;11(1):97–100.
3. Kennedy DN, O'Craven KM, Ticho BS, Goldstein AM, Makris N, Henson JW. Structural and functional brain asymmetries in human situs inversus totalis. *Neurology.* 1999;53(6):1260–1265.
4. Bates JI, Netsky MG. Developmental anomalies of the horns of the lateral ventricles. *J Neuropathol Exp Neurol.* 1955;14(3):316–325.
5. Wilson M. *The anatomical foundation of neuroradiology of the brain.* Boston, MA: Little Brown; 1963.

6. Achiron R, Yagel S, Rotstein Z, Inbar O, Mashiach S, Lipitz S. Cerebral lateral ventricular asymmetry: is this a normal ultrasonographic finding in the fetal brain? *Obstet Gynecol*. 1997;89(2):233–237.

7. Shen EY, Huang FY. Sonographic finding of ventricular asymmetry in neonatal brain. *Arch Dis Child*. 1989;64(5):730–732.

8. Geschwind N, Levitsky W. Human brain: left-right asymmetries in temporal speech region. *Science*. 1968;161(3837):186–187.

9. Wada JA, Clarke R, Hamm A. Cerebral hemispheric asymmetry in humans. Cortical speech zones in 100 adults and 100 infant brains. *Arch Neurol*. 1975;32(4):239–246.

10. Rubens AB, Mahowald MW, Hutton JT. Asymmetry of the lateral (sylvian) fissures in man. *Neurology*. 1976;26(7):620–624.

11. Gannon PJ, Holloway RL, Broadfield DC, Braun AR. Asymmetry of chimpanzee planum temporale: humanlike pattern of Wernicke's brain language area homolog. *Science*. 1998;279(5348):220–222.

12. Heilbroner PL, Holloway RL. Anatomical brain asymmetries in New World and Old World monkeys: stages of temporal lobe development in primate evolution. *Am J Phys Anthropol*. 1988;76(1):39–48.

13. Chiu HC, Damasio AR. Human cerebral asymmetries evaluated by computed tomography. *J Neurol Neurosurg Psychiatry*. 1980;43(10):873–878.

14. Weinstein S. Functional cerebral hemispheric asymmetry. In: Kinsbourne M, ed. *Asymmetrical function of the brain*. Cambridge, UK: Cambridge University Press; 1978:40.

15. Brain WR. *Speech disorders*. London, UK: Butterworth; 1961.

16. Kinsbourne M, ed. *Asymmetrical function of the brain*. Cambridge, UK: Cambridge University Press; 1978.

17. Schenker N. Microstructural asymmetries of the cerebral cortex in humans and other mammals. In: Hopkins, WD, ed. *The evolution of hemispheric specialization in primates*. London: Academic Press; 2007.

18. Bodian D. Discussion. In: Mountcastle VB, ed., *Interhemispheric relations and cerebral dominance*. Baltimore, MD: Johns Hopkins Press; 1962:25–26.

19. Muckli L, Naumer MJ, Singer W. Bilateral visual field maps in a patient with only one hemisphere. *Proc Natl Acad Sci USA*. 2009;106(31):13034–13039.

20. Jeelani NU, Jindahra P, Tamber MS, Poon TL, Kabasele P, James-Galton M, Stevens J, et al. Hemispherical asymmetry in the Meyer's Loop: a prospective study of visual-field deficits in 105 cases undergoing anterior temporal lobe resection for epilepsy. *J Neurol Neurosurg Psychiatry*. 2010;81(9):985–991.

21. Catani M, Mesulam M. The arcuate fasciculus and the disconnection theme in language and aphasia: history and current state. *Cortex*. 2008;44(8):953–961.

22. Nathan PW, Smith MC, Deacon P. The corticospinal tracts in man. Course and location of fibres at different segmental levels. *Brain*. 1990;113(Pt 2:303–324).

23. Huna-Baron R, Landau K, Rosenberg M, Warren FA, Kupersmith MJ. Unilateral swollen disc due to increased intracranial pressure. *Neurology*. 2001;56(11):1588–1590.

24. Maxner CE, Freedman MI, Corbett JJ. Asymmetric papilledema and visual loss in pseudotumour cerebri. *Can J Neurol Sci*. 1987;14(4):593–596.

25. Hayreh SS. The sheath of the optic nerve. *Ophthalmologica*. 1984;189(1-2):54–63.

26. Bartley AJ, Jones DW, Weinberger DR. Genetic variability of human brain size and cortical gyral patterns. *Brain*. 1997;120 (Pt 2):257–269.

27. Thompson PM, Cannon TD, Narr KL, van Erp T, Poutanen VP, Huttunen M, Lönnqvist J, et al. Genetic influences on brain structure. *Nat Neurosci*. 2001;4(12):1253–1258.

13

Decussation

Neurologists regularly encounter a hemiparesis caused by a contralateral cerebral lesion. We seldom pause to ponder the origin of this crossed pattern. Ideas about this subject vary, with some believing that the visual system was the original site of crossing and others favoring the spinal cord.

Much of the discussion of crossed wiring deals with the optic chiasm. In fish, there is total crossing; the fibers from one eye project to the contralateral side of the brain. At first glance, the human system seems totally different. The homonymous hemianopsia due to a unilateral occipital lesion demonstrates that input from both eyes is received by each occipital lobe. However, humans retain a remnant of the total crossing pattern of fish. The *monocular temporal crescent* is the term we use for the totally crossed portion of the visual field of each human eye. Retinal fibers from the most anteronasal portion of the retina are those that totally cross.

Speculation began with Ramòn y Cajal.[1] He took an interest in the total crossing of the visual system of fish and other lateral-eyed animals. He suggested that crossing of vision was necessary because the lens of each eye inverts its image. Crossing, he thought, brought the two inverted images into a continuous panorama in the brain. He considered the crossing of vision as primary. This idea was expanded upon by Vulliemoz. He reasoned that a visual stimulus to the left of a fish would be detected by the right brain. In turn, the right brain could activate the ipsilateral rubrospinal and vestibulospinal pathways. These ipsilateral motor pathways could activate the right-sided axial musculature, allowing the fish to coil away from the left-sided stimulus.[2]

Kinsbourne proposed a 180-degree somatic twist hypothesis to account for decussation of the chiasm. His idea is that decussation itself may have conferred no evolutionary advantage. He suggests that decussation is merely a byproduct of a twist of the ventral nervous system of the invertebrate to form what became the dorsal system of the vertebrate. If this twist to a dorsal nervous system conferred some evolutionary advantage, the associated crossing of the optic nerves would have been secondary.[3]

An alternative hypothesis of the crossed chiasm has been suggested.[4] A symmetric ancestor of vertebrates could have, for some reason, rolled 90 degrees onto its left side and thereby lost symmetry with the vertical midline. For an active swimmer, there could have been an evolutionary advantage to regaining this symmetry, to again have the two sides of the body to the right and left of the vertical. de Lussanet states that return to symmetry could have occurred in one of two ways, either by a 90-degree turn back to the original vertical or by a further 90-degree turn in the direction of the initial turn to the left, thereby fully inverting the original body position.

De Lussanet suggests that both of these possible compensations occurred.[4] Remember, the ancestor turned on its left side. Regaining symmetry, they propose, occurred when the anterior head turned another 90 degrees in the same direction while everything caudal to the head, including the midbrain and mouth, turned 90 degrees in the opposite direction, toward the original swimming position. "As a result the rostral head region in the adult vertebrate is twisted and inverted with respect to the caudal body parts."[4] The eyes and the forebrain are now inverted, but their sites of connection are not. In other words, retinal axons must now cross to get to their formerly ipsilateral intended targets in the thalamus and tectum. Their explanation for crossing of the trochlear nerve from the midbrain to the contralateral superior oblique muscle is analogous to the chiasmal crossing theory, but there is no satisfactory reason in this theory for the third and sixth cranial nerves retaining ipsilateralconnections.

Commentary on the decussation of vision continues. Other speculations about the origin of decussation have been offered.[5] It has been observed that it was the abandonment of the fully crossed visual system which enabled enabled primates to develop stereopsis at arm's length.[6]

Right-to-left crossing, however, did not necessarily originate with vision. Very reasonable is the concept of Sarnat and Netsky that crossed connections were basic to the spinal cord of an ancestor of the vertebrates. The ancient coiling reflex is triggered by external stimulation. The sensory input via interneurons stimulates contralateral spinal cord motor neurons, allowing an ancestor to coil away from the stimulus. In addition, swimming required crossing interneurons that would allow "alternating contraction of myotomes on the two sides of the body."[1] In evolution, they posit, the crossed spinal connections would have preceded any visual crossing. Once crossing was established at the spinal level, it may have set a pattern of crossing that was carried through evolution of higher centers.

CLINICAL ASPECTS

The visual fields of the two eyes overlap greatly. Beyond this binocular field, each eye has a temporal crescent, a peripheral "crescent moon"-shaped portion of the field, which is detected in only one eye and is projected to only the contralateral hemisphere. The temporal crescent is represented in the anterior 10% of the primary visual cortex and is seen in the far 60–90 degrees of the visual field. This remnant of the totally crossed visual field of the fish has been very useful to the clinician over the years. Detection of a temporal crescent field defect in one eye has been a clue to a contralateral anterior occipital lesion.[7] Sparing of the temporal crescent in an occipital lobe infarct has suggested that the lesion is posterior.

Detection of defects in or sparing of the temporal crescent have been described as an endangered finding because current methods of visual field testing do not show enough of the visual field to display the crescent.[8] Manual kinetic perimetry and Goldmann visual fields showed the temporal crescent well. Today, automated static perimetry dominates; this method typically does not display the peripheral field well. Thus, the temporal crescent cannot be studied by this method.

Once invaluable in the pre-computed tomography/magnetic resonance imaging (CT/MRI) scan era, visual fields are now less essential to localize lesions. The automated methods are designed for study of glaucoma not cerebral disease. Although the temporal crescent is not often examined today, the neurologist must know of it, that a one-eye complaint can be due to a contralateral cerebral lesion. Furthermore, the neurologist must know that homonymous hemianopsia can be perceived as a one-eyed problem because the temporal field defect (with involvement of the crescent) is bigger in one eye than the nasal field defect in the other eye.

LACK OF TYPICAL CROSSING

There are long-lived humans who lack standard chiasmal crossing patterns. Those with albinism, for example, have a greater percentage of crossed fibers at the chiasm than do non-albinos.[9] Furthermore, healthy humans can lack a chiasm altogether. Humans with normal visual fields can have achiasma with see-saw nystagmus.[10] See-saw nystagmus is the clue to achiasma in Belgian sheepdogs.[11]

One can survive very nicely with an uncrossed upper motor neuron pathway. This atypical anatomy has been nicely documented in some patients with congenital mirror movements.[12] Absence of a pyramidal decussation can also be seen in Klippel-Feil syndrome, in X-linked Kallmann's syndrome, and in other congenital diseases.[2] Terakawa used functional MRI and sensory evoked potentials to study a case of hemiparesis ipsilateral to a putaminal hemorrhage.[13] Hosokawa used MRI to demonstrate ipsilateral Wallerian degeneration of the corticospinal tract in a patient with an old thalamic hemorrhage and ipsilateral hemiplegia.[14] The uncrossed pyramidal tract had been well-documented by the autopsy study of Verheart and Kramer.[15] The neurologist must know about the possibility of an uncrossed corticospinal tract in order to understand the rare patient with a hemiparesis ipsilateral to a stroke.

Upper motor neuron pathways from the left cerebral hemisphere mediate not only voluntary movements of the right side of the body but also turning of the head to the right. It is the left accessory nerve that causes the left sternocleidomastoid muscle to contract and turn the head to the right, but it has been a puzzle as to how the typically decussating upper motor neuron pathway would signal the ipsilateral accessory nerve to coordinate the head movement to the right. (Such connections are well known to mediate eye movements. Voluntary gaze to the right requires the left cerebral hemisphere to send a message to the left third cranial nerve nucleus. These eye movement connections are relatively well understood.) Similarly, the message descending from the left cerebrum must get to the left cervical motor neurons, which give rise to the accessory nerve. The specific connections that tell the sternocleidomastoid muscle to contract are not clear, and the experiments of Bender are not reported in enough detail for us to draw any conclusions.[16] Geschwind suggested several possible anatomical explanations.[17]

The neurologic findings of a cerebellar lesion are uncrossed on the body. This ipsilateral pattern results from a double crossing. The cerebellum projects to the contralateral motor cortex via the superior cerebellar peduncle and brachium conjunctivum. Cerebellar modulation of the contralateral cortical motor area shows its effect ipsilateral to a cerebellar lesion because the corticospinal tract crosses as it descends in the medulla oblongata.

The crossed relationship of cerebellum and motor cortex has long been known from the occurrence of crossed cerebellar atrophy. An old unilateral cerebral lesion can result in contralateral cerebellar atrophy. The crossed relationship of cerebrum and cerebellum also can be seen in vivo. MRI scans can show reversible increased signal on fluid-attenuation inversion recovery (FLAIR) MRI in the cerebellar hemisphere contralateral to a cerebral focus of repeated seizures. These remote physiologic effects are referred to as crossed cerebellar diaschisis.[18-20]

CONCLUSION

The presence of crossed neurological systems is basic to clinical neurology. Crossing, however, appears to not be essential. One can survive without an optic chiasm. One can do nicely with an uncrossed corticospinal tract. When there is crossing, the amount of crossing can vary from individual to individual. We can track across vertebrate species the evolution of complete chiasmal crossing to the diminished crossing seen in the human visual system. This change in crossing of vision is very understandable as a correlate of the evolution of a lateral-eyed animal to a frontal-eyed human. The origin of crossing cannot be determined with certainty. We can only speculate about how many times crossing developed in pre-vertebrate history or what advantages, if any, crossing conferred. As clinicians, however, we do have to be prepared to recognize patients with uncrossed anatomy—a challenge when we expect systems to be crossed as usual.

REFERENCES

1. Sarnat HB, Netsky MG. *Evolution of the nervous system.* New York: Oxford University Press; 1974.
2. Vulliemoz S, Raineteau O, Jabaudon D. Reaching beyond the midline: why are human brains cross wired? *Lancet Neurol.* 2005;4(2):87–99.
3. Kinsbourne M, ed. *Asymmetrical function of the brain.* Cambridge: Cambridge University Press; 1978.
4. De Lussanet MHE, Osse JWM. An ancestral axial twist explains the contralateral forebrain and the optic chiasm in vertebrates. *Animal Biol.* 2012;62:193–216
5. Loosemore RG. The inversion hypothesis: a novel explanation for the contralaterality of the human brain. *Biosci Hypotheses.* 2009;2(6):375–382.
6. Larsson M. The optic chiasm: a turning point in the evolution of eye/hand coordination. *Front Zool.* 2013;10(1):41.
7. Shenkin HA, Leopold IH. Localizing value of temporal crescent defects in the visual fields. *Arch NeurPsych.* 1945;54(2):97–101.
8. Lepore FE. The preserved temporal crescent: the clinical implications of an "endangered" finding. *Neurology.* 2001;57(10):1918–1921.
9. Guillery RW, Okoro AN, Witkop CJ. Abnormal visual pathways in the brain of a human albino. *Brain Res.* 1975;96(2):373–377.
10. Apkarian P, Bour LJ. See-saw nystagmus and congenital nystagmus identified in the non-decussating retinal-fugal fiber syndrome. *Strabismus.* 2001;9(3):143–163.
11. Dell'Osso LF. See-saw nystagmus in dogs and humans: an international, across-discipline, serendipitous collaboration. *Neurology.* 1996;47(6):1372–1374.
12. Brandão P, Jovem C, Brasil-Neto JP, Tomaz C, Descoteaux M, Allam N. Congenital mirror movements: lack of decussation of pyramids. *Brain.* 2014;137(Pt 8):e292.

13. Terakawa H, Abe K, Nakamura M, Okazaki T, Obashi J, Yanagihara T. Ipsilateral hemiparesis after putaminal hemorrhage due to uncrossed pyramidal tract. *Neurology*. 2000;54(9):1801–1805.

14. Hosokawa S, Tsuji S, Uozumi T, Matsunaga K, Toda K, Ota S. Ipsilateral hemiplegia caused by right internal capsule and thalamic hemorrhage: demonstration of predominant ipsilateral innervation of motor and sensory systems by MRI, MEP, and SEP. *Neurology*. 1996;46(4):1146–1149.

15. Verhaart WJC, Kramer W. The uncrossed pyramidal tract. *Acta Psychiatr Neurol Scand*. 1952;27(1–2):181–200.

16. Bender MB, Shanzer S, Wagman IH. On the physiologic decussation concerned with head turning. *Confin Neurol*. 1964;24:169–181.

17. Geschwind N. Nature of the decussated innervation of the sternocleidomastoid muscle. *Ann Neurol*. 1981;10(5):495.

18. Strefling AM, Urich H. Crossed cerebellar atrophy: an old problem revisited. *Acta Neuropathol*. 1982;57(2–3):197–202.

19. Kozić D, Kostić VS. Crossed cerebrocerebellar atrophy. *Arch Neurol*. 2001;58(11):1929–1930.

20. Fantaneanu TA, Tang V, Lum C, Guberman A. Epilepsy and crossed cerebellar diaschisis with persistent cerebellar syndrome. *Can J Neurol Sci*. 2012;39(1):87–88.

14

Lowly Origins

Human neuroanatomy carries a record of our vertebrate ancestors, and neurologic disease also reveals traces of human evolution. Neurology is more understandable and more interesting when the clinician is attuned to our ancient neurological circuits. Much of the thinking about this subject is speculative.

NERVES

The wrap-around course of the radial and peroneal nerves is intriguing. Synthesizing what is known about limb evolution, we can make conceptual sense of this anatomy. Precursors of the arm and leg are the sprawling limbs of the primitive tetrapod. They extend laterally. By evolution, the limbs come to elevate the body off the ground. More importantly for our subject, the forelimbs rotate 90 degrees posteriorly and the hindlimbs rotate 90 degrees anteriorly into positions relatively close to the body. Thereby, in the quadruped mammal, the elbow and knee face each other. In the anterior limb, a superimposed forward torsion allows the paws to be aligned anteriorly (Figure 14.1). In this process of rotation and torsion, the radial nerve, in maintaining connection to its antigravity muscles, ends up wrapping around the humerus. The wrapping of the peroneal nerve around the fibula undoubtedly also develops from rotation and torsion as the pelvic fin evolves into the modern mammalian hindlimb. There is remarkably little written about peripheral nerve evolution.

With the emergence of bipedalism, the abdominal contents and fat are pulled by gravity toward the legs. The gravity vector has been changed by about 90% from that of the tetrapod.[1] The weight of this sometimes pendulous mass can severely compress the lateral femoral cutaneous nerve. Had we remained on four legs, we would not have been vulnerable to this mononeuropathy.

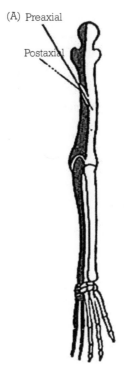

(A) Preaxial

Postaxial

FORELIMB

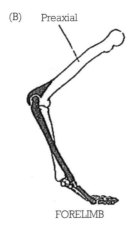

(B)   Preaxial

FORELIMB

Figure 14.1 (A) The bones of the forelimb of a primitive tetrapod with the postaxial aspects of the limb bones darkened. Through evolution, rotation and torsion of the limb result in changed relationships of the bones, seen in the mammal forelimb (B). This rotation and torsion is associated with changes in muscles and nerves. Humans manifest the demonstrated effects of this limb evolution. (From Flower's *An Introduction to the Osteology of Mammalia*, 1885.)

The original appearance of the brachial and lumbosacral plexi cannot be placed. Sharks, as ancient as they are, already have multiple nerve roots going to each fin, and these nerves merge and divide in a complicated pattern. When several myotomes merged into a fin, the muscle segments were admixed and the associated nerves meshed into networks.[2] With the evolution of limbs from fins, our brachial and lumbosacral plexi have become even more complex.

SPINE

Cervical and lumbar disorders account for much of clinical neurology. The bony spines of the nonhuman primates and newborn humans maintain the fundamental mammalian shape, an arch. In bipedal humans, however, the spinal arch develops into a sinuous structure. This single vertebral column supports much of the body mass, with lumbar lordosis allowing the trunk to be balanced over the hips and cervical lordosis allowing the vertebral column to support the mass of our remarkably enlarged brains. Furthermore, the neck and lumbar spine become much more mobile in the bipedal human than in other primates. The wear and tear from this mobility and weight-bearing causes humans to suffer with neck pain, back pain, and radiculopathy.

Radiculopathy due to intervertebral disc herniation reminds us that the nucleus pulposus is a remnant of the notochord. When we are embryos, vertebrae largely replace this cartilaginous, axial rod, which is a characteristic of all vertebrates. The clinical neurologist can encounter the remnants of notochord in ways other than disc herniation. When the annulus fibrosis degenerates, vascular connections allow embolism of fibrocartilaginous fragments, with resulting spinal cord infarctions.[3] Because the vertebral column and clivus are derived from the notochord, it is along this skull base–spine axis that chordomas occur. In occasional individuals, there is a notochordal rest within a vertebral body. Such remnants of the notochord can connect two intervertebral discs. These rests, when large, can be mistaken for chordomas unless diffusion-weighted sequences are included on magnetic resonance imaging (MRI).[4] On computed tomography (CT) scans, calcified remnants of the notochord sometimes can be seen in the midline between the clivus and the posterior wall of the nasopharynx.

LOCOMOTION

Bipedal locomotion carries neurologic implications other than spinal disease. The quadrupeds, including the nonhuman primates, usually move about on four limbs. The support of four limbs is much more secure than the support of two. For the biped, stability is much more vulnerable to a loss of sensation, vision, or vestibular or cerebellar function. We take advantage of this relative instability when we check for a Romberg sign or look for difficulty with tandem gait. Bipeds are also vulnerable to blood pressure dropping when they rise. Orthostatic hypotension is not a problem for alligators.

When some polio victims with withered legs learned to crawl, observation of these patients led to speculation that this quadrupedal gait was like that of a chimpanzee; that is, an emergence of an evolutionarily more ancient form of locomotion. Careful study has shown that this idea was incorrect. Humans with weak legs use a lateral sequence gait like that of a baby crawling. The lower primates use a diagonal sequence gait. Thus, human crawling is not a manifestation of an older primate gait mechanism.[5]

GILLS

The human embryo never develops gills. However, the outpouchings of the oropharyngeal tube and gill arches appear just as they do in fish. These branchial (gill) arches have evolved into many important structures that persist in humans. In addition, the central neural circuitry that controlled the pumping of water through the gills probably manifests itself in humans.

Bony derivatives of gill arches include the hyoid, mandible, and middle ear bones. Cranial nerves that supply gill arches survive in humans as the trigeminal, facial, glossopharyngeal, vagal, and accessory nerves. Gill arch musculature survives as our muscles of facial expression and mastication.[6] These ancestral relationships have been clearly traced by study of comparative anatomy and human embryology. Does the physiology, the neurologic circuitry related to gills, survive in humans? Scholars hypothesize that disease can reveal vestigial mechanisms for pumping water through gills. Palatal tremor and hiccoughs have been discussed. Stern reasoned as follows:

> The significance of rhythmic palatopharyngeal myoclonus (RPM) has remained obscure. The movements resemble superficially quick deglutition in which the palate, uvula, pharynx, base of tongue and larynx cooperate to close off the respiratory passages against aspiration. The net effect of the repeated movements is to create a rhythmic reciprocating expansion and contraction of the oral cavity with corresponding relative negative and positive pressures.
>
> In the vertebrates oropharyngeal dynamics of this type would fit best with the needs of the gill breathers such as fish and amphibian larvae. The

oxygen bearing water is drawn continually into the mouth by enlargement of the oral cavity and forced out over the gills through the gill slits and opercula by contraction of the oropharynx. All of these structures function in continuous synchronous reciprocating rhythm. The expanding and contracting phases there correspond to the expanding and constricting phases of RPM.

On the basis of the similar oropharyngeal dynamics, the hypothesis can then be set forth that rhythmic palatopharyngeal myoclonus is the human homologue of a primitive accessory respiratory reflex in gill-breathing vertebrates.[7]

Yakovlev later concurred that palatal myoclonus (palatal tremor, palatopharyngeal myoclonus, or palatal nystagmus) was a manifestation of an ancestral gill pumping movement:

Now the rhythmic myoclonus is, in contrast to random myoclonus, a much more clear-cut and consistent anatomico-clinical syndrome. It affects with distinct predilection the musculature of branchial derivation, the soft palate, the larynx, the pharynx and the facial and jaw musculature. . . . The muscular contractions are eminently rhythmic and the rhythm is usually slow, in the range of from 20 to 60 per minute. The synergic contractions of branchial muscles persist in sleep unaltered in their rhythm or rate. The rhythmical myoclonus of the branchial musculature . . . is a release phenomenon.[8]

Review of respiratory control in fish is compatible with this hypothesis. In most teleosts, the respiratory rate is of 60–100 per minute, a rate in the range of palatal myoclonus.[9] The oscillating larynx (laryngeal myoclonus) is a related phenomenon of similar rate.[10]

Hiccoughs are the subject of further speculation. The rhythmic contractions of pharyngeal muscles pump water through the gills of premetamorphic tadpoles. After the gills atrophy, the tadpoles use lungs for breathing. Nevertheless, the rhythmic contractions of the buccal cavity persist. To prevent aspiration during this phase of development, there must be rhythmic glottis closure. It has been suggested that human hiccoughs, with their repetitive contractions and glottis closure, are due to a related, residual brainstem circuit because hiccoughs also occur in lower mammals.[11] Furthermore, the occurrence of human hiccoughs in utero indicates that there is an inborn motor pattern for them.

EYES

In the lateral-eyed fish, each eye projects a different view of the world to the brain. The images do not overlap. Vestibulo-ocular reflexes stabilize the images when a fish rolls a bit from side to side or swims up or down. This image stabilization is accomplished by the appropriate movement of the extraocular muscles. The recti muscles, for example, play this role when the fish tilts right or left. Image stabilization can be considered the "ancient and original function of the eye muscles."[12]

With evolution, the human sees the world with frontal eyes, and the visual field of each eye overlaps with the other. In addition, insertions and angles of action of the extraocular muscles change. These modifications have implications for the clinical neurologist.

The fused overlapping visual fields of our bifrontal eyes give us the advantage of stereopsis at arm's length. However, bifrontal eyes make us vulnerable to diplopia. If an extraocular muscle is very weak, the eyes are misaligned and their images cannot be fused. A lateral-eyed fish or rabbit does not have this problem.

Although vestibulo-ocular reflexes may not be as critical to humans as to lateral-eyed animals, "they are still the first line of defense when the head moves" (David Zee, MD, by email, 2016). Furthermore they are very useful to the neurologist. In the comatose patient, we use them routinely to test the function of extraocular muscles and their cranial nerves. In addition, we recognize that skew deviation indicates a disturbance in vestibulo-ocular and related posterior fossa circuitry.[13] (In the lateral-eyed fish, skew deviation is normal when the animal tilts to the side.)

The angle of action of the superior oblique muscle has changed so greatly that it is practically unnecessary for eye movement in the human.[14] Nevertheless, it remains useful to the neurologist who is examining a patient with an oculomotor nerve palsy. Attempted depression of the eye when it is fully adducted causes a torsional movement that informs the neurologist that the trochlear nerve and its nucleus are intact.

Although the extraocular muscles have changed their orientation to the axis of the eye, and although not all of these muscles are as important as they once were, the extrinsic muscles of the human eye have otherwise changed little from those of the shark. They are similar in appearance and consistent in innervation. They are perhaps the best conserved muscles in all of vertebrate evolution.[15] Development of limbs, loss of gills, assumption of bipedal locomotion, and development of a huge brain has had virtually no effect on these muscles. The extraocular muscles and their neural control are truly, in Shubin's term, our "inner fish."[16]

Of course, one could argue that the eye itself deserves this title. The sun radiates a large range of frequencies, of which visible light is but a small part. Visible light is the portion of the electromagnetic spectrum that is least attenuated by seawater. In other words, the vertebrate eye evolved in response to the photons that penetrated the world of the ancient fish. Since X-rays or radio waves did not make their way into the ancient ocean, our piscine ancestors had no opportunity to respond to their frequencies, and we, the descendants, are blind to them. As our ancestors did, we look out through salty water—our tears, which bathe our corneas and allow us to see.

REFERENCES

1. Latimer B. The perils of being bipedal. *Ann Biomed Eng.* 2005;33(1):3–6.
2. Hyman LH. *Comparative vertebrate anatomy.* 2nd ed. Chicago: University of Chicago Press; 1942.
3. Bots GT, Wattendorff AR, Buruma OJ, Roos RA, Endtz LJ. Acute myelopathy caused by fibrocartilaginous emboli. *Neurology.* 1981;31(10):1250–1256.
4. Oner AY, Akpek S, Tali T, Ucar M. Giant vertebral notochordal rest: magnetic resonance and diffusion weighted imaging findings. *Korean J Radiol.* 2009;10(3):303–306.
5. Lanska DJ. A human quadrupedal gait following poliomyelitis: from the Dercum-Muybridge collaboration (1885). *Neurology.* 2016;86(9):872–876.
6. Herrick CJ. The criteria of homology in the peripheral nervous system. *J Comp Neurol Psychol.* 1909;19(2): 203–209.
7. Stern MM. Rhythmic palatopharyngeal myoclonus, review, case report and significance. *J Nerv Ment Dis.* 1949;109(1):48–53.
8. Yakolev PI. Discussion of Luttrell CN, Bang FB. Myoclonus in cats with Newcastle disease virus encephalitis. *Trans Am Neurol Assoc.* 1956;(81st Meeting):59–64.
9. El-Mallakh RS. Branchial myoclonus: the expression of archaic respiratory gill movements in man? *J Theoret Neurobiol.* 1987;5:153–159.
10. Plummer C, Vogrin S, Cook M, Moses D. Curing of oscillating larynx by levetiracetam. *Arch Neurol.* 2011;68(8):1075. doi:10.1001/archneurol.2011.168.
11. Straus C, Vasilakos K, Wilson RJA, et al. A phylogenetic hypothesis for the origin of hiccough. *Bioessays.* 2003;25(2):182-18.
12. Walls GL. The evolutionary history of eye movements. *Vision Res.* 1962;2;69–80.
13. Zee DS. Considerations on the mechanisms of alternating skew deviation in patients with cerebellar lesions. *J Vestib Res.* 6(6):395–401.
14. Simpson JI, Graf W. Eye-muscle geometry and compensatory eye movements in lateral-eyed and frontal-eyed animals. *Ann N Y Acad Sci.* 1981;374:20–30.
15. Gilbert PW. The origin and development of the human extrinsic ocular muscles. *Contrib Embryol.* 1957;36:59–78.
16. Shubin N. *Your inner fish: a journey into the 3.5-billion-year history of the human body.* New York: Pantheon Books; 2008.

15

Learning Neurology

L earning neurology is a lifelong process. As one begins to learn neurology, he or she acquires basic facts and approaches. Simplified concepts of anatomy and pathology facilitate the initial stages of learning, but at some point in the process one advances by learning that nervous system, anatomy, diseases, and phenomena vary greatly.

Even the most basic concept that we learn is a simplification. There is, for example, the division of neuronal processes into two types, axons and dendrites. This distinction is "based upon an idealized nerve cell, exemplified by the mammalian ventral horn motor neuron."[1] Having acquired this concept, the neurologist can eventually learn that reality is more complex. Amacrine cells of the retina and granule cells of the olfactory bulb are examples of central nervous system (CNS) cells that lack recognizable axons or dendrites. The dorsal root ganglion cell has central and peripheral processes, both of which act like axons. Further differing from the basic model is the presence of axoaxonal and dendro-dendritic synapses.

Textbooks explain that the part of the optic tract that carries information about the upper visual field sweeps forward in the temporal lobe before turning back toward the occipital lobe. This Meyer's loop is schematically and accurately drawn, but it is a simplification in the sense that it does not indicate that the loop varies from person to person. In one individual, the loop may come more anteriorly than in another.[2] Epileptologists and neurosurgeons performing temporal lobe resection for epilepsy must be aware of these differences. Preoperative diffusion tensor tractography may help predict the likelihood of a postoperative visual field defect.[2]

Other gross anatomic features vary from brain to brain. Occipital lobe surface morphology is a good example.[3] The standard drawing of occipital lobe anatomy gives the student only the basic idea. In reality, the calcarine fissure can be nearly vertical or almost horizontal. The calcarine sulcus terminates by dividing into two rami in more than half of brains. In about 30% of brains, the calcarine sulcus meets the lunate sulcus only after reaching the hemisphere's superolateral surface. The lunate sulcus is highly varied in shape, and standard drawings do not capture these brain-to-brain variations.

Similarly, the superolateral surface of the cerebrum shows variations in morphology.[4] Study of 100 hemispheres showed that the superior frontal sulcus, the superior temporal sulcus, the inferior frontal sulcus, the precentral sulcus, and the postcentral sulcus were discontinuous in 40–70% of hemispheres. The neurologist comes, with growing experience, to realize that the pattern of cerebral sulci varies greatly from the stylized diagrams that orient the beginner to the subject.

Variations occur in the brachial plexus as well. The "normal" anatomy occurs in fewer than half of the cases. For example, the T1 root did not contribute in more than a quarter of cases, and, in some instances, the C4 and T2 roots are part of the formation.[5] Learning "normal" anatomy is adequate for a beginner, but it does not suffice for a more advanced doctor. The electromyographer or neurosurgeon always should be aware of this variability, which can have clinical consequences.

Distally, in the peripheral nervous system, we find similar variability. The standard separateness of the median and ulnar nerves is well known, and learning this pattern is basic neurology. Eventually, however, the electromyographer must learn the variations. Some fibers that initially run with the median nerve may, in varying patterns, cross over to the ulnar nerve. The beginner need not know this, but the specialist in peripheral nerve disease must (Figure 15.1).

Learning is facilitated by good visual display, and some diagrams are more correct; some are easier to absorb. Depending on the learner's level, a simpler or a more complicated diagram will be most helpful. Very often the best diagrams show more than one aspect or variation of the subject (see Figures 15.2–15.8).

HELPING OTHERS LEARN

The first step in teaching is to figure out what you want the students to know and why. With these objectives clear, everything else will follow. Of course, one must know the capacity of the students. Do not try to teach more than a pupil can learn. Remember that it's not what you teach, it's what they hear. It is what gets through that counts. To get something across, the teacher must apply the fundamental pedagogical principle, repetition.

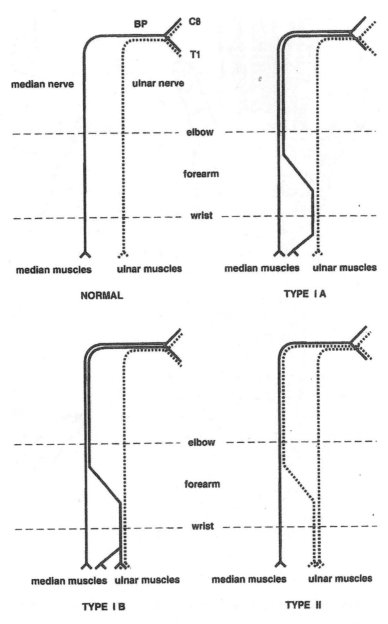

Figure 15.1 Median to ulnar crossover patterns compared with the "normal" anatomy. (From *Focal Peripheral Neuropathies* by John D. Stewart, 4th edition, 2010.)

(A)

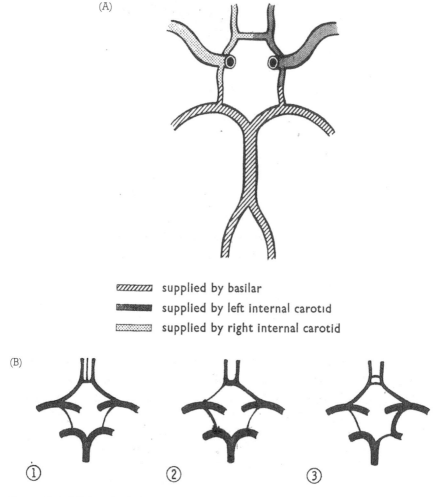

▨▨▨▨ supplied by basilar

▬▬▬▬ supplied by left internal carotid

▨▨▨▨ supplied by right internal carotid

(B)

①   ②   ③

Figure 15.2 (A) Standard idealization of the circle of Willis. (B) Instructive illustration of some varieties of circle of Willis anatomy. (From *The Anatomical Foundation of Neuroradiology of the Brain*, by McClure Wilson, 1963.)

The resident, like the teacher, is ordinary clay. Our goal is to mold the resident into a competent neurologist. Thus, we cannot too often teach how to elicit and recognize the manifestations of upper motor neuron disease. It is most important to emphasize the basics. We can elaborate obscure aspects of a subject. We can expound on history, chemistry, epidemiology, and more. But, in the end, we must return to basics. Repetition is the master word.

Although patient demonstration is central to clinical neurologic education, the lecture also can be effective. It is important to arrive early when you are to lecture. A speaker with a knack for it can engage the audience with humor.

(A)

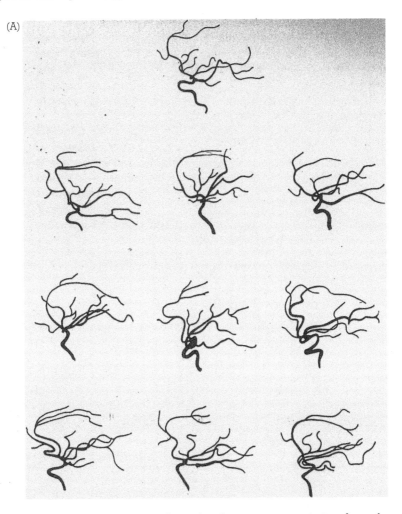

Figure 15.3 Instructive drawings indicate that there are many varieties of vascular supply. (A) varieties of carotid artery supply. (B) Varieties of deep cerebral venous drainage. (From *The Anatomical Foundation of Neuroradiology of the Brain*, by McClure Wilson, 1963.)

In response to a laudatory introduction, James Corbett might say, "My mother would have smiled. My father would have believed it."

In the course of a lecture, one should not simply read projected slides. The audience can read more quickly than the speaker can read aloud. If such slides are necessary, it is better for the speaker to let the audience read while he elaborates on what is projected. Part way through a lecture, it is often helpful to pause, saying: "To summarize so far. . . ."

(B)

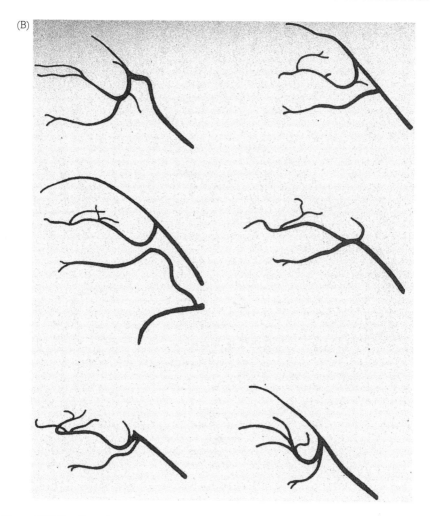

Figure 15.3 Continued

Be yourself. Entertainment of one kind or another can keep the audience alert. Those gifted at mimicry can demonstrate movement disorders, gaits, and forms of dysarthria; those not adept should avoid attempting it. The flamboyant Ben Kean often asked his audience questions. When a resident would call out the correct answer, Kean would pull a cigar from his jacket pocket and fling it as the prize. This kind of showmanship can be memorable; but only those with flair should attempt it.

People like to hear a story, and an audience can follow a story. Thus, whether describing a case or the development of knowledge of a subject, tell it as a story. Keeping the audience attentive is not enough. The main points must be reiterated. Regardless of one's style, it helps to occasionally pause to give the impression of thought. It is important to end a lecture early—never late.

(A)

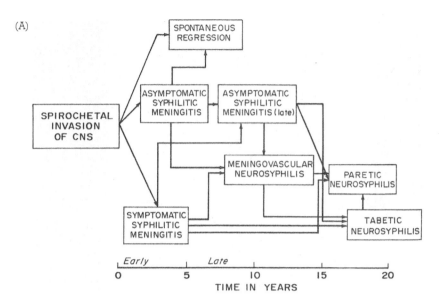

(B)

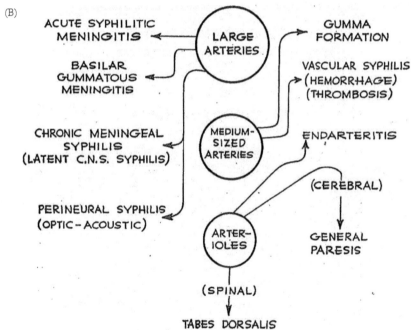

Figure 15.4 Diagrams about neurosyphilis. (A) The concept of the disease as a meningitis. It also shows temporal relationships of clinicopathologic syndromes. This diagram is a superior multifaceted display. (From *Principles of Neurology*, by Adams and Victor, 1977.) (B) A very different concept of neurosyphilis as a vasculitis of different sized arteries. It makes no chronologic correlation. It portrays meningitis as unrelated to, not as the cause of general paresis or tabes dorsalis. (From *Pathology of the Central Nervous System*, by Courville, 3rd edition, 1950.)

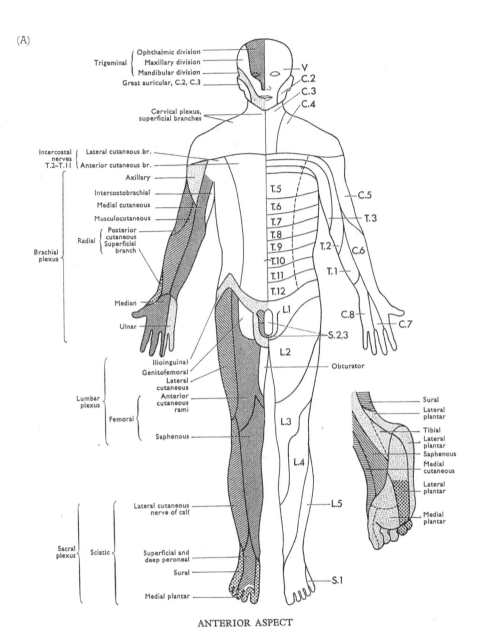

ANTERIOR ASPECT

Figure 15.5 (A) Idealized map of the areas of sensory supply of nerve roots and nerves. This diagram is so dense with information that it is better for reference than learning. (B) Foerster's instructive display shows that the dermatomes of adjacent nerve roots overlap. Compare to (A), which does not show the overlap.

(B)

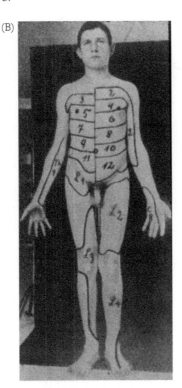

Figure 15.5 Continued

Not every talk should follow the same format. Edward Tufte recommends the method of Jeff Bezos: start a meeting by giving the audience a page or a paper to read. When you begin to speak, you have an already involved audience. Right off, you can comment and expand on what the group has already read. The Socratic method is often helpful. Eventually, however, the teacher must come to a nonconversational exposition.

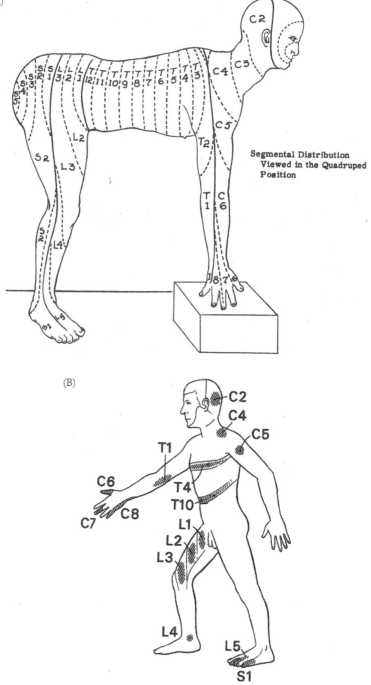

Figure 15.6 Alternate dermatome maps aid learning. (A) helps one learn dermatomes by displaying the human in a quadruped position. Compare to Figure 15.5A. (From *Correlative Neuroanatomy and Functional Neurology*, 12th edition, by Chusid and McDonald, 1964.) (B) helps one learn the utility of dermatomes by simplification. It demonstrates only the signature areas. Compare to Figure 15.5A. (From *Segmental Neurology*, by John K. Wolf, 1981.)

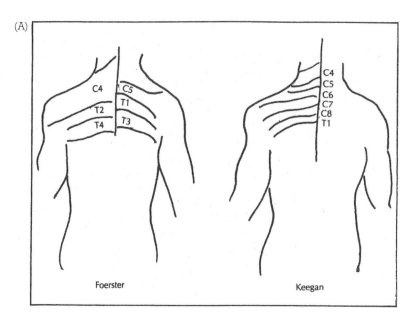

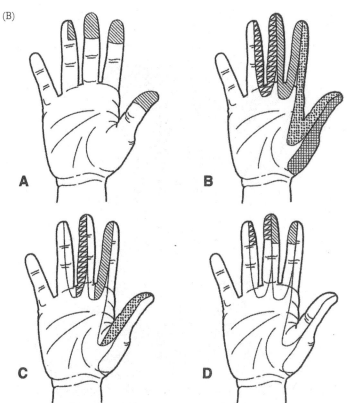

Figure 15.7 Multifaceted diagrams aid learning. (A) Compares the concepts of
dermatomes of two different authors. (B) demonstrates how individuals vary in the
sensory supply of the median nerve. Compare to Figure 15.5A. (From *Focal Peripheral
Neuropathies,* by John D. Stewart, 4th edition, 2010.)

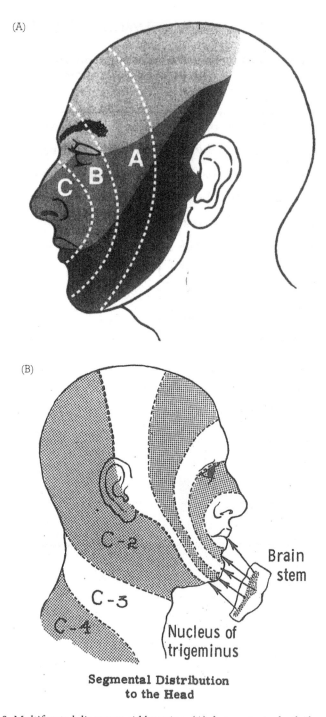

(A)

A

B

C

(B)

C-2

C-3

C-4

Brain
stem

Nucleus of
trigeminus

**Segmental Distribution
to the Head**

Figure 15.8 Multifaceted diagrams aid learning. (A) demonstrates both the sensory supply of trigeminal nerve branches (by shading) and the sensory supply of different regions of the trigeminal nerve nucleus (by concentric rings). (From *How to Examine the Nervous System*, by R. T. Ross, 1969.) (B) Correlates the concentric rings with a drawing of the brainstem. (From *Correlative Neuroanatomy and Functional Neurology*, by Chusid and McDonald, 12th edition, 1964.)

FINAL THOUGHTS

1. We cannot anticipate which statements will hit home with a student. We can only hope that something that we utter will affect his future thinking or put him on a path of study.
2. Teaching the same young doctors during a 3-year residency allows one to address some basic topics repeatedly. Do not hesitate to do it. Repetition is the fundamental pedagogical principle.

REFERENCES

1. Peters A, Paley SL, deF Webster, H. *The fine structure of the nervous system: neurons and their supporting cells.* 3rd ed. New York: Oxford University Press; 1991.
2. Taoka T, Sakamoto M, Nakagawa H, Nakase H, Iwasaki S, Takayama K, Taoka K, et al. Diffusion tensor tractography of the Meyer loop in cases of temporal lobe resection for temporal lobe epilepsy: correlation between postsurgical visual field defect and anterior limit of Meyer loop on tractography. *AJNR Am J Neuroradiol.* 2008;29(7):1329–1334.
3. Mandal L, Mandal SK, Dutta S, Ghosh S, Singh R, Chakraborty SS. Variation of the major sulci of the occipital lobe: a morphological study. *Al Ameen J Med Sci.* 2014; 7(2):141–145.
4. Gonul Y, Songur A, Uzun I, Uygur R, Alkoc OA, Caglar V, Kucuker H. Morphometry, asymmetry and variations of cerebral sulci on superolateral surface of cerebrum in autopsy cases. *Surg Radiol Anat.* 2014;36(7):651–661.
5. Uysal II, Seker M, Karabulut AK, Büyükmumcu M, Ziylan T. Brachial plexus variations in human fetuses. *Neurosurgery.* 2003;53(3):676–684; discussion 684.

16

Selected Concepts

Neurological concepts come and go. Some endure and some evolve. Some are disproved and some are ignored. With new methods, data, and ideas, fresh concepts emerge. In this chapter, we examine several neurologic concepts that illustrate this flux in neurological thinking.

TRANSIENT ISCHEMIC ATTACK

C. Miller Fisher brought attention to the subject of transient ischemic attacks (TIA) at the second conference on cerebrovascular disease at Princeton, in January 1957.[1] The terminology was not fixed. He also referred to TIAs as transient ischemic episodes or transient attacks. Such attacks had been known before Fisher's paper, but little attention had been paid to them. They had been alternately attributed to vasospasm or episodic arterial hypotension (Figure 16.1).

In the volume that included Fisher's paper, there was appended a report of an ad hoc committee appointed through the National Institutes of Health. The document was a classification and outline of cerebrovascular diseases. In this report, prepared by Fisher, Raymond Adams, and others[2], the term TIA was avoided. TIAs were referred to as "transient cerebral ischemia without infarction" or "recurrent focal cerebral ischemic attacks." In short order, however, the term TIA was widely adopted. Over the subsequent years of discussion, there was general recognition that most TIAs last less than 1 hour. Nevertheless, focal attacks lasting up to 24 hours were included in the definition of TIA in a 1975 revision of the classification of cerebrovascular disease.[3]

New methods of stroke imaging and acute stroke therapy brought increasing attention to TIA and its definition. Neuropathologists had long known that some brain infarcts are asymptomatic and that some are transiently

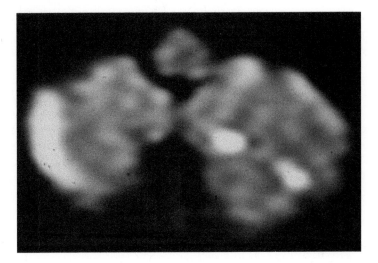

Figure 16.1 This patient briefly experienced ataxia. By the old definition, he had a transient ischemic attack (TIA). By the new definition, the acute infarcts seen on magnetic resonance imaging exclude the diagnosis of TIA.

symptomatic. That clinical transience does not equate to pathologic transience became obvious to every neurologist in the era of computed tomography (CT) and magnetic resonance imaging (MRI) scanning. Hence, in 2009 multiple national organizations endorsed a new definition of TIA: "a transient episode of neurological dysfunction caused by a focal brain, spinal cord or retinal ischemia, without acute infarction."[4] In effect, this definition means that a TIA is transient episode of ischemia for which the brain MRI shows no correlate.

When C. Miller Fisher proposed the term "transient ischemic attack," Raymond Adams told him, "It will never fly". (C. Miller Fisher, MD, in conversation, 2007). Fisher's term succeeded in that it has been widely adopted, and it has been clinically useful for more than half a century.In a sense however, Adams had been right. Adams was as much a neuropathologist as a neurologist. By the old definition, TIA was heterogeneous in its neuropathology. With the new definition, Adams would likely be comfortable. He would readily accept the concept of TIA that is now based on the state of the brain as revealed by modern imaging.

REFERENCES

1. Fisher CM. Intermittent cerebral ischemia. In: Wright IS, Millikan CH, eds. *Cerebral vascular diseases.* New York: Grune & Stratton; 1958; 81–98.

2. Laureno R. *Raymond Adams: a life of mind and muscle*. New York: Oxford University Press; 2009.

3. Albers GW, Caplan LR, Easton JD, Fayad PB, Mohr JP, Saver JL, Sherman DG, et al. Transient ischemic attack--proposal for a new definition. *N Engl J Med*. 2002;347(21):1713–1716.

4. Easton JD, Saver JL, Albers GW, Alberts MJ, Chaturvedi S, Feldmann E, Hatsukami TS, et al. Definition and evaluation of transient ischemic attack: a scientific statement for healthcare professionals from the American Heart Association/American Stroke Association Stroke Council; Council on Cardiovascular Surgery and Anesthesia; Council on Cardiovascular Radiology and Intervention; Council on Cardiovascular Nursing; and the Interdisciplinary Council on Peripheral Vascular Disease. *Stroke*. 2009;40(6):2276–2293.

THORACIC OUTLET SYNDROMES

A clinical syndrome is a constellation of signs and symptoms; it is a recognizable entity. In this sense, thoracic outlet syndrome (TOS) is not a syndrome at all. It is a term applied to various conditions. Furthermore, TOS does not affect the thoracic outlet, which by classical anatomical terminology is the thoracic aperture at the diaphragm. Nevertheless, this term has been widely used for more than half a century since Rogers[1] and then Peet[2] popularized it. There was resistance, however, and Sunderland refused to use the term in his encyclopedic text.[3] Resigned to the prevalent use of the term, Gilliat found the plural form, "thoracic outlet syndromes," less objectionable.[4]

Because the term TOS had become pervasive, Asa Wilbourn clarified it by offering a definition: "a collective term, describing a number of disorders attributed to compromise of blood vessels and/or nerves at any of several points between the base of the neck and the axilla."[5] This comprehensive definition includes a spectrum of ischemic disorders of the arm due to compression of the subclavian and/or axillary arteries and a spectrum of disorders of venous insufficiency of the arm due to compression of the subclavian or axillary vein. This definition also includes neurologic compromise in this region. The neurologic manifestations arise from stretching of the C8–T1 roots or the lower brachial plexus over a fibrous band, arising from a rudimentary cervical rib or an elongated C7 transverse process and extending to the first rib.[6] Typical features are thenar atrophy and pain and paresthesias in the medial aspect of the arm. Ulnar sensory nerve action potentials are decreased in amplitude.

This classification of TOS into arterial, venous, and neurogenic problems in the cervicobrachial region was reached after a century of confusion. In the early decades, the label TOS was applied to patients with other neurologic conditions. Before cervical radiculopathy and carpal tunnel syndrome were discovered, many patients with these problems were thought to have TOS. Once neurologists had become knowledgeable about median nerve entrapment and cervical root compression, they rarely diagnosed neurogenic TOS.

For certain vascular surgeons, however, the idea that neurogenic TOS was very common persisted.[7] They inappropriately took an interest in patients with nonvascular arm symptoms and came to believe that various arm symptoms were due to a form of TOS even when there was no cervical rib or elongated cervical transverse process. Because they were the doctors who operated on arterial TOS and venous TOS, they believed they could successfully intervene in nonvascular cases. Their reports prolonged the confusion about neurogenic TOS in the general medical community, and they performed unnecessary surgery by the hundreds at certain hospitals. This epidemic of unnecessary surgery began to abate a few decades ago.

A more recent cause of confusion about TOS was the application of the term to compressive neuropathies, such as those due to the prolonged wearing of a back pack. This loose use of terminology has not helped clarify the often confusing topic of TOS.

True neurogenic thoracic outlet syndrome is real but much less common than carpal tunnel syndrome or cervical radiculopathy. The work of Roger Gilliat and writing of Asa Wilbourn have clarified this subject for neurologists.

REFERENCES

1. Rogers L. Upper-limb pain due to lesions of the thoracic outlet; the scalenus syndrome, cervical rib, and costoclavicular compression. *Br Med J.* 1949;2(4634):956–958.
2. Peet RM, Henriksen JD, Anderson TP, Martin GM. Thoracic-outlet syndrome: evaluation of a therapeutic exercise program. *Proc Staff Meet Mayo Clin.* 1956 May 2;31(9):281–287.
3. Sunderland S. *Nerve and nerve injuries.* London, UK: Churchill Livingstone; 1968.
4. Gilliatt RW. Thoracic outlet syndromes. In: Dyck PJ, Thomas PK, Lambert EH, eds., *Peripheral neuropathy*, 2nd ed. Philadelphia, WB Saunders;1984:1409–1424.
5. Wilbourn AJ. Thoracic outlet syndrome. In: *AAEE course D: radiculopathies.* Rochester, MN: American Association of Electromyography and Electrodiagnosis; 1989:28–38.
6. Gilliatt RW, Le Quesne PM, Logue V, Sumner AJ. Wasting of the hand associated with a cervical rib or band. *J Neurol Neurosurg Psychiatry.* 1970;33(5):615–624.
7. Wilbourn AJ. Thoracic outlet syndrome is overdiagnosed. *Muscle Nerve.* 1999;22(1):130-6-7.

UNCAL HERNIATION

Mass effect from a unilateral cerebral hemisphere lesion can lead to brainstem dysfunction. Ipsilateral oculomotor nerve involvement, especially dilatation of the pupil, often heralds the onset of coma. Autopsy of such causes often shows a groove in the uncus, indicating that, as a part of this process, the medial temporal lobe has been pushed from the middle cranial fossa, over the edge of the tentorium toward the midbrain. This uncal herniation has been considered the main event in the clinical deterioration of cerebral mass lesions. In this concept, the dilatation of the pupil has been attributed to third-nerve compression by the medial temporal lobe as it passes over the tentorial edge.

All of these observations—the mass effect, the pupil dilatation as a harbinger of coma, and the uncal grooving from herniation—were never doubted. It was the causal linkage that was questioned as early as the first edition of *Principles of Neurology*. Adams and Victor were "more impressed with the functional importance of the lateral than downward displacement."[1] Adams's colleagues at the Massachusetts General Hospital pursued this subject. Fisher studied calcified pineal glands on CT head scans and concluded that the cerebral mass lesions primarily caused lateral shifting, not downward movement.[2] Ropper studied another 24 patients by CT scans with a more quantitative analysis.[3] He found that the early anatomic manifestation of decline in consciousness was due to horizontal, not downward, displacement. He supported his conclusions with subsequent quantitative measurements on MRI scans.[4]

In a later review, Fisher would sum up by saying that "temporal lobe herniation is not the means by which the midbrain sustains irreversible damage."[5] "Lateral displacement of the brain at the tentorium is the prime mover and herniation a harmless accompaniment."[5] As a corollary, the dilated pupil is attributed to midbrain distortion instead of uncal herniation.

Although temporal lobe herniation is an epiphenomenon and not the main process responsible for the decline into coma, the term "herniation" survives. It seems to be ensconced in medical jargon

REFERENCES

1. Adams RD, Victor M. *Principles of neurology.* New York: McGraw Hill; 1977.
2. Fisher CM. Observations concerning brain herniations. *Ann Neurol.* 1983;14(1);100.
3. Ropper AH. Lateral displacement of the brain and level of consciousness in patients with an acute hemispheral mass. *N Engl J Med.* 1986;314(15):953–958.

4. Ropper AH. A preliminary MRI study of the geometry of brain displacement and level of consciousness with acute intracranial masses. *Neurology.* 1989;39(5):622–627.

5. Fisher CM. Brain herniation: a revision of classical concepts. *Can J Neurol Sci.* 1995;22(2):83–91.

DISCONNECTION SYNDROMES

Geschwind's "disconnection syndromes" was his term for what his 19th-century predecessors' called "conduction disorders." Presumably by analogy with electrical circuits, white matter tracts were thought to conduct messages from one cortical area to another. Before World War I, impaired conduction in such circuits was the model for many higher cortical disorders. The diagrams of postulated connections became so complex that Henry Head mocked them, and a decline in work on conduction models followed the war.

At mid-century, Norman Geschwind was becoming the American most knowledgeable about the European literature on aphasia, agnosia, and apraxia. His lengthy essay in the journal *Brain* discussed the anatomic work of Paul Flechsig, the experimental animal work of Sperry and colleagues, and human case reports and case series, especially from the continental literature. His two-part paper renewed interest in conduction disorders, now under the term "disconnection syndromes."[1,2] Some authorities were skeptical.[3] With the advent of MRI scanning, it became obvious that a simple disconnection model could not explain all aphasias and their lesions.[4]

Those seeking circuits to explain higher cerebral functions have found that brains are more variable and complicated than we would like. During the second half of the 20th century, Geschwind's astute writings and lectures stimulated interest in the subject of higher cortical disorders, but his models have proved inadequate.

On the 40th anniversary of the publication of Geschwind's well-known article, Catani and Hytche wrote that concepts of hyperconnectivity and cortical hyperactivity were needed to supplement disconnection theory.[5] On the 50th anniversary of Geschwind's paper, Mesulam discussed the legacy of the disconnection concept. He explained that, to some extent, the concept of networks has replaced a simple concept of connection and disconnection.[6] With the network concept, a new wave of diagram-making is emerging.

In discussing localization and aphasia, Raymond Adams doubted that a simple answer would be found. He stated, "We cannot even strictly work out the localization of the movement of the hand." Understanding the neurophysiology of higher cortical function, he implied, is likely to be more difficult (Raymond Adams, MD, in conversation, 2005).

REFERENCES

1. Geschwind N. Disconnexion syndromes in animals and man. I. *Brain.* 1965;88(2):237–294.
2. Geschwind N. Disconnexion syndromes in animals and man. II. *Brain.* 1965;88(3):585–664.
3. Crichley M. Notices of recent publications. *Brain.* 1975;98(4):723.
4. Willmes K and Poeck K. To what extent can aphasia syndromes be localized? *Brain* 1993;116:1527–1540.
5. Catani M. and Hytche D. The rises and falls of disconnection syndromes. *Brain* 2005;128:2224–2239.
6. Mesulam MM. Fifty years of disconnexion legacy. *Brain* 2015;138:2791–2799.

WILBRAND'S KNEE

Wilbrand's knee,[1] a neuropathologic observation, gave rise to a concept that was unquestioned for most of the 20th century.[1] The concept was that decussated retinal fibers detour into the contralateral optic nerve before they enter the optic tract and that this detour is responsible for a particular pattern of visual field loss in parasellar lesions. Wilbrand propounded that a lesion affecting the inferonasal optic nerve near the chiasm could cause not only an ipsilateral optic nerve visual field defect, but also a superior temporal defect in the field of the contralateral eye. This superior temporal field loss he attributed to fibers that made the detour into the opposite, compressed optic nerve. Wilbrand called this pattern the "anterior chiasmal syndrome," although the putative lesion was in the optic nerve.

Wilbrand's knee was long-lived as a concept because it was such a neat anatomical–clinical correlation and because it could be usefully applied at the bedside. The sophisticated observer could recognize that this combination of field defects was not be due to an anterior optic nerve lesion but was due to a lesion of the optic nerve near the chiasm.

Wilbrand, however, had discovered these detoured fibers in a case of long-standing unilateral enucleation.[1] He saw the knee only in the atrophic optic nerve of the enucleated eye. The pathological material showed a detour (knee) of 1–2 mm.[1,2] Nevertheless, he later exaggerated the extent of the knee to 5 mm, and he portrayed the detoured fibers as a normal feature of the anterior visual pathway (Figure 16.2).[1,3]

With the advent of modern anatomic methods, Jonathan Horton was able to study the subject of Wilbrand's knee in two species of monkeys. He performed uniocular injection of radioactive proline in normal monkeys. At autopsies done at different intervals, he was able to trace the retinal axons from the injected eye.

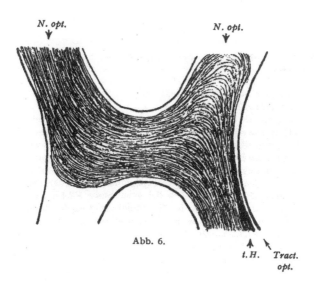

Abb. 6.

N. opt.

N. opt.

t. H.   Tract. opt.

Figure 16.2 Wilbrand's drawing of his concept that fibers from one optic nerve, after decussation, detour into the contralateral optic nerve.

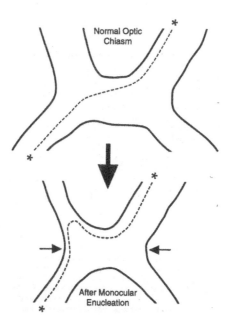

Normal Optic Chiasm

After Monocular Enucleation

Figure 16.3 Horton's drawing compares the decussation of the normal state with that after monocular enucleation of long standing. (From Horton JC. Wilbrand's knee of the primate optic chiasm is an artifact of monocular enucleation. *Trans Am Ophthalmol Soc.* 1997;95:579–609. Republished with permission of the American Ophthalmological Society.)

There was no evidence for Wilbrand's knee. He then did experiments after enucleation of one eye. A few months after enucleation, he injected the tracer into the remaining eye. At autopsy, the radioactive amino acid revealed no knee. However, when he injected the normal eye years after unilateral enucleation, autopsy did reveal Wilbrand's knee in the atrophic optic nerve on the side of the enucleation. In other words, Wilbrand's knee is not normal anatomy. It is an artifact seen in long-standing enucleation-related optic atrophy (Figure 16.3).

The development of MRI has improved the study of patients with the "anterior chiasmal syndrome." The common cause of this visual field pattern is pituitary adenoma affecting the chiasm as well as the optic nerve. Study of tuberculum sellae meningioma patients with similar visual fields also shows chiasmal involvement.

In sum, the concept that Wilbrand's knee is normal anatomy and the related ideas about its relationship to visual fields have been disproved. The concept has not withstood the scrutiny of modern methods in the hands of an able, patient, and thoughtful scientist. There can be death pangs for beloved concepts. When I attended a lecture at which Jonathan Horton presented his data, a prominent neurosurgeon erupted in protest. It was hard for the learned man to give up a clever concept that he had diligently memorized and repeatedly taught.

REFERENCES

1. Horton JC. Wilbrand's knee of the primate optic chiasm is an artefact of monocular enucleation. *Trans Am Ophthalmol Soc.* 1997;95:579–609.
2. Wilbrand H., Saenger A. *Die Neurologie des Auges.* Wiesbaden: J. Bergmann; 1904: vol. 3, part I, 98–120.
3. Wilbrand H., Schema des Verlaufs der Schnervenfasern durch das Chiasma. *Z Augenheilkd* 1926;59:135–144.

NEWER CONCEPTS

Over the past half century, we have witnessed great technological advances. Newer scientific methods, such as MRI scanning, have led to new knowledge that has necessitated changes in neurologic concepts. During recent decades, new concepts have emerged. Infectious proteins, antibody-mediated brain disease, channelopathies, and the glymphatic system are relatively new ideas. We cannot foresee how our understanding of these concepts will be advanced or modified in the coming decades.

INDEX